NUTRITION

CW01073059

MENOPAUSE

HOW YOUR DIET CAN HELP

Stephen Terrass

Thorsons
An Imprint of HarperCollins*Publishers*

*To Nicola, whose love, understanding, patience,
encouragement and valuable input have helped me
immeasurably in the writing of this book.*

Thorsons
An Imprint of HarperCollins*Publishers*
77–85 Fulham Palace Road,
Hammersmith, London W6 8JB
1160 Battery Street,
San Francisco, California 94111-1213

Published by Thorsons 1994
10 9 8 7 6 5 4 3 2 1

A catalogue record for this book
is available from the British Library

ISBN 0 7225 2985 6

Printed in Great Britain by
HarperCollinsManufacturing, Glasgow

CONTENTS

ACKNOWLEDGEMENTS

The author wishes to thank the following for their valuable support and assistance in this project: Richard Passwater, Ph.D. for his inspiration, and for providing the Foreword and reviewing the manuscript; editor Sarah Sutton and copy-editor Barbara Vesey; special thanks to Rand Skolnick, John Steenson, Cheryl Thallon and Leyanne Scharff for their valuable support; and Nibs Laskor for his help and generosity. Most of all, fondest thanks to Nicola Squire and Shirley Terrass for their love and encouragement.

As a young male researcher studying nutrition, I had little concept of the importance of its role in menopause. In 1974, however, I surveyed approximately 9,000 women on their use of vitamin E. The survey questionnaire contained no questions about nor any suggestion of menopause, yet women took the time and effort to voluntarily relate their dramatic experiences as to how vitamin E, along with magnesium and calcium, turned their unbearable situations into virtually no problems at all. I was so impressed with these dramatic stories that I published them in *Prevention* magazine in 1976.

I always watch the scientific literature for studies involving the role of nutrition in menopause. In 1991 I published a chapter in *The New Supernutrition* relating the newer information on the subject, and I have received hundred of letters from women who were helped by improved diets and nutritional supplements. Thus, I know that they work and that the advice given in this book works. Stephen Terrass's approach is based on the latest scientific and medical research. It has been adapted for the needs of the individual thanks to his personal experience in counselling and the 'feedback' he has had from his lectures on the subject.

Stephen Terrass is sensitive to the physical and

emotional consequences of menopause. Although neither the author nor myself can experience the suffering that some women endure, we do understand the problem. And we have both experienced the joy of being told by women of the difference our nutritional advice has made. Stephen Terrass provides excellent and well-researched advice on the role of diet and nutritional supplements including herbs. He explains what is happening during menopause and why it is happening, to help you understand the process, then looks at the pros and cons of conventional and complementary medical therapies and the role of nutrition in easing the journey through menopause. Advice is also given on protecting yourself against osteoporosis, heart disease and other disorders that have been linked to the menopause.

The benefits of the advice given in this book extend well beyond the 'change of life' itself to produce life-long better health.

Richard A. Passwater, Ph.D.
February 1994

The human body is a very mysterious and fascinating organism. When we observe the function and purpose of each system in the body, it is clear that most everything is so logical, yet so complex. These complexities exist in both sexes; nevertheless a special mystery enshrouds the very unique and special capabilities of women.

One area which is a great problem for women, however, (biologically speaking), is the fact that a particularly intricate balance in body chemistry must be maintained in order for optimal health to be achieved. This is not exclusive to women; the biochemistry of both women *and* men is balanced on a knife edge. However, the balance that needs to be struck in a woman's body appears to be infinitely harder to maintain.

Perhaps the area where this problem shows up the most is in the female reproductive system. By reproductive system we are not merely referring to the system whereby a woman can bear children. As you will find out, the female reproductive system also accounts for many aspects of a woman's health: physical, mental and emotional. The same reproductive system which allows a woman to have children is actually inextricably linked to systems in her body with entirely different functions and purposes.

Perhaps the best analogy for this precise and dependent relationship is to imagine something being suspended from a chain. The entire purpose and function of this chain – and each of its links – is completely dependent on *all* the others carrying out their tasks. If even one link is incapable of fulfilling its purpose properly, the suspended object crashes to the ground. Now, this analogy is obviously a blatant over-simplification of the functioning of a woman's body. Nevertheless there is a pertinent comparison to be made. In a chain each link has the exact same function. In the human body, each 'link' has a different function; but the overall purpose and goal is the same for each link in the body – to keep the body alive and in peak condition.

From the time that a girl reaches puberty, she goes from having physical and biological characteristics which resemble those of the opposite sex to being greatly different. Adolescence also happens to be the time when the hormonal changes reminiscent of adulthood begin to manifest. A girl gradually becomes a 'woman', from both an emotional and a physical point of view. The changes which begin to occur at this point will remain more or less in place for many years to come.

With the changes which bring about the onset of sexual adulthood comes a young girl's ever-increasing awareness of her body. A new undercurrent of impulses are brought on due to the surge in hormones. Feelings of sexuality, increased awareness of self-esteem, increased feelings of responsibility, control and direction – all these can begin to flourish in a very distinct and positive manner at this time, and most are attributable, directly or indirectly, to the biochemical changes that are taking place.

A decade or so down the line, a woman often chooses to fulfil one of the primary physiological purposes of these hormones – to have a child. If this stage occurs, the next several years are spent nurturing offspring. Of course, if you have children yourself you have probably already realized that this stage actually never ends! At any rate, later on in life a woman reaches a point when her body has spent its resources for 'species propagation'; she begins the last major change – the end of the reproductive process, which is called the *menopause*.

Menopause is often spoken of as if it were a disease! To be honest, considering the experience that many women go through at this time, no one could blame them for classifying it this way. Nevertheless, the menopause is far from a disease. It is a normal and predetermined change which happens in all women.

While you will be aware of the changes that happen to a girl beginning menstruation, the menopause causes changes of its own. Actually, in many aspects the two stages are more or less diametrically opposed to one another, and as such many of the physical processes of each are a sort of reverse of the other. Basically, one process readies the body for the purpose of fertility and its underpinnings; the other process signals a weakening of that same infrastructure.

This process is initiated by a reversal of the hormonal pattern found in puberty. Hormones, especially oestrogen, account not only for reproductive capabilities but also for the changes to and onset of maturity in a girl's physical appearance when she is going through puberty. The opposite is true of the menopause, as the depletion of these hormones is manifested by a steady reduction of what we think of as certain 'female' characteristics. These changes are not only experienced in a physical manner, however. There are many emotional and mental consequences for women as well.

By no means do *all* women go through a terrible time at this stage, but many women will know all too well about the negative changes associated with the onset of the menopause. Hot flushes, a lack of energy, vaginal dryness, severely irregular periods, reduction in the tightness of the skin, depression, forgetfulness and many other symptoms can accompany this stage. In addition, for many women these changes are not occasional occurrences but become chronic at this time.

Like menstruation, the menopause is a very personal matter. Only women who have experienced the changes themselves can fully understand what they are like, and it is this which leads to some of the greatest stress attributed to this time of life. As many of the symptoms of such hormonal changes remain more or less 'invisible' to husbands, children, friends, etc., it is less likely that the menopausal woman will receive all the understanding that she rightly deserves. As a result, a woman may spend much of her time suffering quietly without much support or acceptance from others. This used to be the case with premenstrual tension (PMT) as well, at least before the high profile of the condition prompted medical and scientific research which proved beyond a shadow of a doubt that PMT definitely *is* real. Although there are still the unfortunate jokes about some women using premenstrual tension as an excuse for being 'difficult' or 'lazy', the truth is far from that and more and more men are coming to terms with this fact. Not fast enough, some women will no doubt say!

Many of the symptoms of the menopause are not often as quick in their onset or as acute in their manifestation as those of PMT, but in some ways they are probably harder to cope with. First of all, PMT has very well known and distinguishable symptoms such as irritability, cramps, weight gain, breast tenderness, depression and mood swings, among others. Menopause can have very distinguishable symptoms as well, but they are probably not as well known. This fact may exacerbate any lack of understanding and support shown by others, especially men. For instance, if a woman has mood swings and her partner knows it is 'that time of the month', then he may be more likely to try to understand these as part of a temporary and uncontrollable phenomenon. If a menopausal woman has mood swings or depression her partner is not as likely to attribute these to the fact that she is, temporarily, at the mercy of hormonal influences.

Secondly, premenstrual symptoms are often fairly consistent in timing from one month to the next. Because of this, they may be easier to prepare for (as if such a thing were possible!) for both the sufferer and others. In menopause there is no way to predict all of the symptoms consistently, as they are not restricted to a predetermined cycle.

Thirdly, because the menopause is not a cyclic disorder *per se*, there may be no respite from its symptoms from day to day for a long time. This incessant suffering may understandably have a dreadful impact on the quality of a woman's life for quite a long time.

One other effect which can occur as a result of menopausal changes is the severe weakening of the bones, known as *osteoporosis*. The consequences of this condition are quite worrying, and if left unaddressed, the problem continues to worsen. The end result can be devastating in many cases. Osteoporosis is certainly proof that the menopause is no joking matter. Its hormonal changes can cause more than just a few hot flushes. Not every woman will suffer greatly as a result of the menopause, but every woman *will* experience some changes as a result of the reduction in hormonal activity. How severe or acute these changes are varies from woman to woman. The better the state of the woman's reproductive system to begin with, and the more gradual the menopausal changes, the better the woman is likely to cope. Regardless of how mild or severe symptoms become for a woman at this time, one thing is certain: even minor suffering is more than any woman should have to bear.

The good news is that there is hope on the horizon for those who suffer greatly throughout the menopause. If we look back to the major research on premenstrual tension, an important and encouraging trend occurred: Not only did the research help explain and verify that such a condition really existed, it also prompted a greater understanding of exactly what factors caused PMT in the first place. This knowledge then led to the formulation of more effective and safer treatments for the disorder. There is certainly no reason to think that the same thing will not happen in the case of the menopause. As a matter of fact, the great controversies over hormone replacement therapy (HRT) and the ever-increasing concerns about osteoporosis have stimulated an aggressive effort on the part of the scientific and medical profession to understand the menopause and its workings much better. Fortunately, a growing amount of this research is occurring in the area of natural medicine. Many of the results of such research has confirmed that there are many natural methods of therapy that have proven benefits in treating the symptoms and causes of the problems associated with the menopause – without the high risk of side-effects.

As has been found with PMT, even significant

volumes of medical and scientific proof will not change the collective attitude of the sceptics overnight. Nevertheless, the process is moving in the right direction. In the meantime, it is vital that menopausal and pre-menopausal women are educated about their situation and how to relieve their suffering. That is the focus of this book, which will explain what goes on in a woman's body at this stage of life; how the hormones work; the general symptoms and causes of the menopause and its problems; and the truth behind the confusion over osteoporosis. We will also discuss the natural and very safe methods that can be used for treating and/or preventing menopausal symptoms and related disorders such as osteoporosis.

Menopause is, without a doubt, one of the most taxing periods in a woman's life. Given a proper understanding of the biochemical changes involved, however, a woman can avoid much of the confusion, desperation and self-blame which may accompany the effect of the menopause on her body, her emotional and mental state, and even on her relationships with those around her. An understanding of what can be done to relieve or even prevent such problems can bring new hope of a menopause without misery!

CHAPTER 1

What is the Menopause?

Many people are under the impression that the menopause is some sort of health disorder. This misapprehension may be in part due to the understandable association of the menopause with premenstrual tension (PMT). While PMT is definitely a disorder, the menopause is a very normal and natural process which will occur in the bodies of all women when they reach a certain point in their lives.

The female reproductive system has three major stages: the development phase, which begins to occur from conception; the fertile stage, which begins at puberty; and the menopausal stage, which occurs after the fertile stage begins to wind down.

The menopausal stage of a woman's reproductive life primarily signifies the point when the *ovaries* (the female sex glands) begin to reduce their production of hormones such as *oestrogen* and the supply of eggs becomes close to being exhausted. As hormones such as oestrogen play a huge role in a woman's fertility, and as eggs are obviously necessary in order to produce offspring, the depletion of both leads to the end of a woman's ability to have children. This process can begin at varying ages in a woman's life, but the average age of onset seems to be between the fourth and fifth decade of life.

Most women are unlikely to mind the waning of fertility which happens at this age, as they may well have had all the children that they wanted – but, as you know, infertility is not the only characteristic of the menopausal stage. The changes in the reproductive system which cause the reduction in fertility account for many different processes in the body – and these processes do *not* always happen slowly enough for the body to adjust easily.

In order to better understand what the menopause is, and how and why it occurs, it is important to take a look at the role of the reproductive system and its hormones.

THE FEMALE REPRODUCTIVE SYSTEM

Obviously, the female reproductive system is the system that makes it possible for a woman to bear a child. It also plays a role in the subsequent nurturing and feeding of the child. All mammals possess a very intricate system whereby they can carry out this miracle of life. Of course, this process cannot happen if there is only a woman involved! Nevertheless, the lion's share of the burden falls (as usual) on the woman. The reproductive 'hardware' (and 'software' for that matter) lies not only within a woman's reproductive organs but within certain other glands of the endocrine system as well. It is this fact that contributes to the great difficulty in either treating or even understanding female reproductive imbalances.

Parts and Substances of the Female Reproductive System

THE PRIMARY REPRODUCTIVE 'HARDWARE' IS MADE UP OF THE FOLLOWING:

- *ovaries*
- *uterus*
- *fallopian tubes*
- *vagina*
- *cervix*
- *follicles*
- *ovum (egg)*

THE REPRODUCTIVE 'SOFTWARE' INCLUDES:

- *pituitary gland*
- *hypothalamus gland*
- *adrenal glands*
- *oestrogen*
- *progesterone*
- *follicle stimulating hormone*
- *(FSH)*
- *luteinizing hormone (LH)*

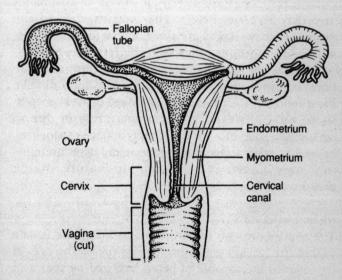

FIGURE 1.1. THE FEMALE REPRODUCTIVE SYSTEM

The Ovaries

The ovaries are the primary sex organs (gonads) in women. They play a major role in the primary processes of reproductive functioning, and as such they are essential in understanding the menopause. As you can see in Figure 1.1. a woman's ovaries are really fairly small. Considering their size, it is difficult to believe that they could play such a major role in the body.

FUNCTION

A primary purpose of the ovaries is the production of the major female reproductive hormones such as *oestrogen* and *progesterone*. These hormones are the prime instigators of the different processes of fertility. The function of the ovaries as well as of the female reproductive hormones are directly involved in a woman's monthly *menstrual cycle*. The ovaries, due to the hormones they secrete, are also essential to many different bodily functions other than the fertility processes. As long as the ovaries are functioning properly, the body can generally maintain a healthy reproductive functioning. If the ovaries are damaged or weakened in some way, however, either prematurely or due to ageing, the state of a woman's reproductive capabilities, as well as other functioning, can rapidly deteriorate. As you may know, this is a major feature of the menopause.

FOLLICLES AND EGGS

The ovaries are also responsible for holding the female half of the fertility equation, the *eggs* (ova). The eggs in the ovaries are capable of being fertilized by sperm in order to create offspring. Each egg is attached to a what is known as a *follicle*. The number of follicles (and thus the number of eggs) contained in the ovaries of a woman vary, depending mostly on her age. While the eggs and follicles in a female infant can number in the millions, by the time puberty arrives there may be less than a half a million. Once this supply of eggs is significantly depleted as time goes on, the chance of fertility becomes less and less. There is a predetermined loss of follicles which occurs as a result of a process called *atresia*. This process eventually leads to an exhausted supply of eggs and follicles, and thus, infertility. Of course, the older you are the greater the extent of the atresia. This is a significant factor in the onset of the menopause.

The Uterus, Fallopian Tubes, Cervical Canal and Vagina

The *uterus* is the organ that carries a developing baby prior to birth. The uterus is very muscular in nature. This muscularity helps to protect the growing baby as well as allowing the baby to be expelled into the *cervical canal* toward the *vagina* at the time of birth.

A special lining called the *endometrium* exists on the walls of the uterus. It is the endometrium which sheds each month during menstruation.

While the cervical canal is primarily a transport vessel for childbirth, the vagina plays a role more specifically related to sex and sexuality. The integrity of the vagina (that is, its texture, size and secretions) during the menstrual years begins to change as the woman moves closer to menopause. The main reason for this is that the reproductive hormones account for certain aspects of the vagina in the first place. As hormonal activity begins to wane, the vagina changes as well.

Once an egg has been released by its follicle, it moves out of the ovary and into the *Fallopian tube*. This tube runs from the ovary to the uterus, and is the area where fertilization of the egg by sperm could take place.

THE COMPUTER INSIDE YOU

Without a doubt, the reproductive 'software' is infinitely more complex and fascinating than the above mentioned parts of the body. The human body is not unlike a high-tech computer in that each cell of each tissue of each organ or gland carries out a pre-programmed command – providing 'the right button is pushed', so to speak. Depending on which command is given, the cells initiate a given bodily process – usually without fail or error. Much like a computer, however, such processes are not guaranteed to be executed perfectly. When cells *do* make a mistake it is not usually because of 'computer error' but because the commands being given are faulty in some way.

The cells are generally reliable provided the commands they receive are correct. So where do these commands come from? Actually, it is the *hormones* that provide the commands which initiate bodily processes, including those of the reproductive system. These are often called 'chemical messengers'.

Oestrogen
The hormone *oestrogen* is one of the most well known of all the chemical messengers. Oestrogen is manufactured primarily by the egg-carrying follicles in the ovaries (after ovulation). Certain levels of this hormone can also be made by the *adrenal glands*. The amounts secreted by the adrenal glands increase as the menopause occurs. There are three different oestrogens: oestradiol, oestriol and oestrone. In order to simplify things I will refer to all three with the general term oestrogen.

FUNCTIONS

Oestrogen is not limited only to having a direct effect on menstruation and fertility. As a matter of fact, oestrogen accounts for almost all of the typical changes in a woman's body after she reaches puberty. Such changes stimulated by oestrogen (oestradiol) include, among others:

- increased breast size
- vaginal characteristics (texture, size, secretions)
- increased pelvis size (allows for child-bearing requirements)
- greater fat deposits (on the hips and thighs, for example)
- growth of endometrium (uterine wall) in the menstrual cycle
- uterine preparation for pregnancy
- bone calcification

As will be seen, oestrogen also plays a role in the calcification of the bones. This may give you some hint as to the connection between the menopause and the development of osteoporosis, or brittle bone disease.

Progesterone

Progesterone (a progestin) plays its largest role after fertilization and during pregnancy, as it is the main hormone involved in the development of the placenta.

FUNCTIONS

In relation to the normal menstrual cycle, progesterone is released along with oestrogen in the second half of the cycle. Among other things it helps oestrogen in the process of stimulating the growth of the smooth muscle tissue (myometrium) of the uterus. Progesterone also stimulates the secretions of the endometrial glands. The variations in breast size during the menstrual cycle can also be caused by variations in progesterone levels.

While oestrogen and progesterone are certainly among the most important hormones of the reproductive system, they are not the *only* ones involved in sending reproductive commands. While understanding a woman's reproductive system would be much easier if all the commands of the reproductive hormones were initiated by the reproductive organs, unfortunately the system is not that simple.

As has been mentioned, the adrenal glands are able to manufacture hormones, including the *sexual steroids* (such as oestrogens and *androgens* [male steroids]). The adrenals can be considered as 'friendly co-workers' rather than as 'hormonal senior managers'. They supply an alternative source of oestrogen which, as you can imagine, takes some of the pressure off the ovaries and the follicles. This function is particularly of use when the ovaries start producing less and less oestrogen, as occurs when a woman is nearing the menopause, and will be discussed in more detail later.

The ovaries are in fact just the 'middle management' of the female reproductive system. The parts of the body that make and pass down the ultimate commands are actually certain glands which could not be much further away from the reproductive centre.

The Pituitary, the Hypothalamus and Gonadotrophins
The glands in question are found in the brain and are called the *pituitary* and the *hypothalamus glands*. These glands serve many different purposes in the human body.

FUNCTIONS

Due to the wide-ranging control that the pituitary gland has, directly or indirectly, on *other* glands in the human body, it is often considered the 'master gland'. As the hypothalamus actually triggers certain hormonal responses of the pituitary, perhaps it should be called 'the master gland's master'!

The pituitary gland is responsible for the release of several hormones, including the *gonadotrophins*: *follicle stimulating hormone* (FSH) and *luteinizing hormone* (LH)

GONADOTROPHINS

Together FSH and LH play a major part in proper reproductive functioning. They are known as *gonadotrophins* because they stimulate the hormonal activity of the primary sex organs (the gonads) – in this case, the ovaries. The processes initiated by these two hormones are rather detailed and lengthy, but we will try to explain them in relatively basic terms.

Luteinizing hormone is what causes a mature follicle to ovulate. It is during the phase after ovulation that follicles in the ovaries produce higher levels of oestrogen. The funny thing is that the hormones being released in the cells surrounding the ovum at this time are actually *androgens*, or male-type hormones! How could this cause oestrogen to be produced? This is where follicle stimulating hormone (FSH) comes into play. FSH actually causes the follicle to mature; it is responsible for the conversion of the aforementioned androgens into oestrogens.

Without the release of these gonadotrophins from the pituitary, a process initially stimulated by the hypothalamus, the necessary ovarian oestrogens would not be produced.

As you can see, even from this rather brief explanation, many different processes must be in proper working order in order to run the female reproductive system, and there must be correct communication and co-operation between the different glands involved.

MENOPAUSE AND REPRODUCTIVE FUNCTIONING

As you might have guessed, the general role of these reproductive components and their related hormones is inextricably linked, in varying degrees, to menopausal causes and symptoms. Let us now put all the information together so that we can get a clearer picture of exactly what is involved in the onset and progression of the menopause.

Onset of Menopause

As mentioned earlier, the menopause signifies the time when certain ovarian functions, such as the production of oestrogen, begin to diminish significantly. This diminished oestrogen production corresponds to the reduction in the number of egg-bearing follicles.

TIMING

The timing of the onset of the menopause varies from woman to woman, but the average appears to fall between the ages of the mid-forties to the early fifties. Some women, however, may experience some of the first signs even while in their late thirties, although fortunately this is less common.

Generally the onset of the menopause is a natural and fairly gradual occurrence, although some women are flung into an unnatural and immediate menopause, usually due to the surgical removal of the ovaries (complete hysterectomy). This will be discussed in more detail later.

While most of the publicity and common knowledge about the menopause surrounds the loss of oestrogen, other hormones are reduced as well, including progesterone. The reduction in such hormones correlates to the reduction and eventual cessation of the menstrual periods. This makes perfect sense when you consider that the purpose of the menstrual period is to serve as a *fertility* cycle. If the reproductive capability is no longer needed, then presumably the hormones which account for fertility are no longer going to be required in the same quantities. This reduction of hormones is genetically intended to occur, and thus you might expect that it should occur in such a way that the body can easily adjust to the changes.

Many women do not go through very bothersome changes and symptoms as the menopause occurs; it is likely that these women have probably been in a fairly balanced reproductive state for some years prior to the onset. This should *not* be such an exceptional accomplishment, but research shows that the percentage of women today who suffer with significant reproductive imbalances in the years prior to the menopause is alarmingly high.

PMT AND MENOPAUSAL TENDENCIES
For instance, premenstrual tension is a perfect example of just what can happen when a woman is experiencing such imbalances in the years preceding the menopause. Statistics suggest that around 30 per cent of women in their thirties suffer with premenstrual tension. PMT is generally a multifaceted condition, but the major

contributor appears to be a (sometimes severe) imbalance in the levels of various hormones. This is not to say that a chronic sufferer of premenstrual difficulties is guaranteed to suffer throughout the menopause, but it only stands to reason that the likelihood is far greater. This is due to the fact that menstrual and menopausal years blend into one another without any separation whatsoever, and we could therefore assume that any propensity towards reproductive system malfunction in earlier life will be carried into the menopausal years as a matter of course.

Without a separation between the menstrual and menopausal years, a woman does not really have the opportunity to benefit from any 'spontaneous' correction of any tendency to hormonal imbalance. After all, since hormones are released by particular glands of the body, any imbalance of such hormones is often due to a malfunction in the gland responsible for releasing the hormone. What can also happen is that a faulty release of one hormone may cause an imbalance in another. This can occur because certain reproductive hormones trigger one another to be 'turned on' or 'turned off'.

With such an intricate and thoroughly dependent relationship existing between such hormones, it is likely that any hormonal and/or glandular malfunctions a woman has in her menstrual years would be carried into the menopause. This connection between PMT and the menopause will be discussed in more detail later.

The onset of the menopause is triggered, generally speaking, by hormonal changes. It is at this time that perhaps the most disturbing element of the menopause begins – its varied and sometimes unpredictable symptoms. The next chapter looks at these many symptoms in detail.

CHAPTER 2

Menopausal Symptoms

As with many other health difficulties, the most common and well-known symptoms of the menopause may *not* be the most destructive aspects of this stage of life. Nevertheless these symptoms, being the most obviously debilitating, are typically the priority of women who are going through the menopause – and nobody could blame them for that!

The symptoms of the menopause may not be as well known as those of premenstrual tension, but there are certainly some which you will have heard about. They also vary greatly from woman to woman, but a list of many of the more common symptoms would include:

- hot flushes
- night sweats
- depression
- irritability
- fatigue
- vaginal dryness and shrinkage
- heart palpitations
- headaches
- sleeplessness
- weight gain

Osteoporosis, another side-effect of the menopause but one that manifests few symptoms, will be discussed later.

As you can see, the above list is fairly comprehensive and, considering its length, it is no wonder that some menopausal women spend a lot of their time feeling terrible! These symptoms are seldom going to dominate a woman's life, but some women can be affected by one or usually more of these symptoms quite frequently.

In the case of PMT, a woman at least knows that the symptoms are likely to be restricted to a certain number of days, followed by a symptom-free stage. This makes the condition at least a little more practical to cope with. Menopause, and thus the symptoms it brings with it, does not run in cycles *per se*; it can be fairly continual – for a matter of years in some cases.

You may have already noticed that several of the symptoms of the menopause also occur in PMT. This connection is no accident, as will be explained below.

Hot Flushes and Night Sweats

Hot flushes are probably the best-known symptom of the menopause. Perhaps this is in part due to the fact that they do not very often occur in conditions other than menopause. Of course, another reason is that they are so common. Even if a woman has a fairly easy path through this time of life, chances are she will experience a hot flush or two.

Hot flushes and night sweats are among the more significant menopausal symptoms in that they represent very 'physical' occurrences. The importance of this is two-fold. First, the menopause is not a 'heavily sign-posted' time of life. Many of its symptoms can be caused by any number of other factors. If anything positive can be said about hot flushes and night sweats, therefore, they can at least help you to know what you are suffering from (i.e., definitely the menopause)! The second significant aspect of this type of symptom is that hot flushes are unlikely to be construed (either by sufferers or others) as being purely psychological. This may seem a small issue, but anyone who has experienced a lack of support or acceptance from others will know just how important this is.

So just what are hot flushes and night sweats, and why do they happen?

HOT FLUSHES AND BLOOD VESSELS

Hot flushes are actually a symptom of a disturbance in the blood vessels of the body. Hot flushes and night sweats appear to be related to a malfunction in the vascular system whereby all of a sudden there is a significant increase in blood flow to the surface of the skin in the upper part of the body, particularly the head. This circulatory anomaly causes redness and flushing as well as the notorious rise in temperature. While this spontaneous process is not continual, it can be quite frequent in many women.

CIRCULATORY AND HORMONAL MALFUNCTION

Hot flushes and night sweats do not mean that the blood circulation is 'too good'. If anything, overall quite the reverse is true; the blood vessels are malfunctioning. If a radiator in your home were to turn up the temperature repeatedly and spontaneously when the room is already warm, only to turn off the heat just as spontaneously, you would experience a mild, externally-produced version of the mechanics of a hot flush.

The trigger for hot flushes and night sweats appears to be related to the disturbance in the levels of oestrogen brought on by changes in the hypothalamus and the pituitary gland. As with all of the following symptoms mentioned, we will look in greater detail later in this book at how this aspect of the condition may be corrected.

Depression

The subject of menopausal depression is a difficult one. On the one hand it can be almost entirely physiological in nature; on the other there is likely to be a non-physiological link as well. Depression in any form is debilitating and self-perpetuating.

Normally, when we think of depression we think of a psychological or emotional condition in which a person is melancholy or 'down', or perhaps emotionally frail. There is no question that this is often the case, but depression can involve many physical manifestations as well.

SYMPTOMS
The following are some of the main clinically recognized aspects of true depression:

- lethargy
- guilt or lack of self-worth
- sleep disorders
- proneness to eat when unnecessary or lack of appetite
- lack of motivation for physical or mental activity
- morbid thoughts
- lack of alertness

Now, just because a woman in her forties or fifties has one or two of these problems, does not mean she is menopausally depressed; nevertheless these are criteria that can be useful in making a diagnosis. In other words, do not disregard these very genuine menopausal symptoms, and if you are visiting your doctor or gynaecologist, be sure to mention them.

As you can see from this list, depression has a wide scope in the areas of life it can affect. During the menopause, hormonal imbalances appear to be responsible for much of the associated depression – but it can also be said that the depression may actually exacerbate the menopausal process as well, hence making the depression even worse: a very vicious cycle indeed!

It is clear that at least part of the problem of menopausal depression is associated with the glandular disturbances which initiate the hormonal changes.

TRANSITIONAL STRESS

Perhaps the more difficult aspect of menopausal depression to deal with is that which is not strictly caused by any direct glandular changes. Menopause is a very difficult time of life for many women to cope with regardless of whether they suffer with severe symptoms or not. Any transition in life is going to be met with at least some resistance, and the menopause is more than just one transition – it is many all rolled up into one.

LOSS OF SELF-ESTEEM

First of all, many women consider the menopause the last major life change that they will undergo. A woman may feel that she is getting older faster, in a manner of speaking, and that because of this she is less 'feminine' . This makes it very difficult to separate the lack of self-esteem that may be associated with 'hormonal depression' from that which is perhaps more 'situational'.

OVERWHELMING DEBILITATION

Secondly, there is depression which is caused by the debilitating and disturbing symptoms and side-effects of the menopausal hormonal changes. For instance, if you cannot sleep, if you are aggravated by persistent hot flushes, if you are tired all the time, or perhaps if your sex life is being adversely affected by vaginal dryness, it is totally understandable that depression might be an end result.

STRAIN ON RELATIONSHIPS

Thirdly, there is the issue of the difficulty that can occur in relationships. It is difficult for men to understand and fully accept the overwhelming control that female reproductive hormones have over a woman's body. This is, in part, due to the fact that men do not undergo hormonal changes of such acuteness and frequency at any time in life. This is especially true with PMT, but would apply to the menopause as well – and perhaps even more so. After all, publicity over the last several years and the frequency of premenstrual symptoms have led many a sceptical man at least to admit that the problem is initiated by physiological occurrences. Where the menopause is concerned, however, there is not so much common knowledge of the wide range of physio-logically induced symptoms; therefore the sufferer may have to deal with a lack of understanding at times. It is no secret to anyone that such a strain on a relationship can lead to significant depression. This is accentuated by the fact that the menopausal transition may last for more than a few years.

It is probably the case that most women who do suffer symptomatically during the menopause will be occasionally or frequently depressed due to a combination of these factors, both physiological and otherwise.

Irritability

Even though depression and irritability almost seem to be opposites, they often occur together in menopause. They are also probably both caused by, and are both a cause of, other menopausal problems.

HORMONAL FLUCTUATION

The irritability of menopause is generally accompanied by nervous tension and anxiety, and these type of symptoms often 'take turns' with the mental and emotional fatigue and apathy that are often experienced at this time of life. This would suggest a sort of 'short circuit', so to speak. This problem of apparently opposite symptoms is related to the difficulty of the glandular system in some women to adjust and compensate in an even and smooth fashion.

The irritability, like the depression, can adversely affect a woman's relationships with her family, friends, co-workers, etc. The more the sufferer understands what is causing the problem, the better she can explain the problem to others. Also she will be less likely to be angry with herself for having the problem in the first place. This realization can help enormously.

Fatigue

It is very difficult to ascertain the actual cause of the fatigue that is associated with the menopause. This is at least partly due to the fact that fatigue is such an ambiguous term in the first place. It appears likely that, in most cases, fatigue is in part related to the hormonal changes which begin to occur, as well as being caused by the overall debilitating effect of the entire menopausal process.

STRESS

The increased level of stress which may be associated with the menopause is perhaps one of the most fatigue-producing factors of all. Stress and the menopause will be covered briefly in the next chapter, but suffice it to say that the aftermath of either acute or chronic stress can be extreme and prolonged fatigue. Of course, tiredness is also a common symptom of depression.

Vaginal Dryness and Shrinkage

As mentioned in Chapter One, oestrogen induces female adult sexual characteristics during puberty. One such characteristic is the enhancement of the size and the secretions of the vaginal area. With this in mind, it is not difficult to understand how shrinkage and dryness of the vagina occurs as a result of menopause. Not all women will suffer greatly with vaginal disorders during and after the menopause, but those whose adrenal glands are impaired in their production of oestrogen will probably be the most susceptible.

SEXUAL DIFFICULTIES

This change creates many unforeseen problems for the sufferer. The changes, and especially the dryness of the lining of the vagina, can cause sexual intercourse to be extremely painful. It can only be guessed just how damaging this could be to the self-esteem of any woman. It also may put strain on sexual relationships.

Many might think that this 'doesn't matter' so much because they may assume that a woman's sex life changes after the menopause anyway. This is an erroneous assumption. Oestrogen is not the hormone responsible for a woman's sex drive. It is the male hormones (androgens) that feed this drive.

Consequently, after the menopause a woman may well want to continue to lead a sex life consistent with that of her pre-menopausal years.

Weight Gain

The issue of menopausally related weight gain is perhaps the most difficult to explain. It is probably due to a combination of factors rather than just one or two. There are far too many variables to cover completely here, but we will very briefly look at a few of the possibilities.

WEIGHT CONTROL AND THE 'SET-POINT'

First of all, it is important to know that each person's weight appears to be controlled by what is called a 'set-point'. Ultimately this set-point refers to the adjusted ratio of calorie metabolism to the requirements of the body. The body, in absolutely every facet, tries desperately to maintain homeostasis – in other words, to maintain the body's normal functioning. Metabolism of calories is no exception. The set-point seems to take charge whenever your intake of calories alters above or below the amount needed to maintain the level that your body is accustomed to. If the calories are reduced (as would be the case if you were on a slimming diet), the metabolism actually *slows down* to compensate for the reduced level of calories. This may seem far-fetched, but it also appears to be true. It also certainly explains why calorie restriction alone does not often work in weight control over the short term. Over the long term it can be more effective, as the set-point for metabolism can very slowly be altered over time.

SET-POINT OF METABOLISM AND AGE

One of the main problems related to menopausal women is that it would appear that the set-point for weight increases as a person gets older (the same could be true of men). As a result it becomes ever-more difficult to obtain and maintain the weight that you might prefer. So just what is it that controls this set-point?

THYROID GLAND AND METABOLISM

The thyroid gland is primarily responsible for the metabolic rate in the body, but it is not the master of its own profession; it, like the ovaries, uterus, breasts, etc. receives its commands from the pituitary and the hypothalamus in the brain. Now, the *specific* connection between the menopause and the glandular set-point is not generally elucidated adequately to draw many helpful conclusions. Nevertheless, considering it is the hypothalamus and pituitary that carry out the lion's share of the responsibility for hormonal changes and triggering, as well as metabolic rate, there may be a connection between the reduced activity of the hypothalamus and pituitary glands (accompanying the end of the fertility cycle) and the change to the body's set-point of weight.

It does appear that the thyroid gland may become somewhat less functional as a person ages. Because this gland has more of a direct control over fat metabolism (not to mention moods, energy levels, etc.), it stands to reason that any reduction in its activity will be met with an increase in body fat levels.

EXERCISE

Exercise represents one of the more effective ways to alter the set-point of the metabolism of calories. If anything, physical activity is likely to decrease as a woman gets older. This, as you can guess, will only make matters worse.

There are, of course, many other symptoms that can be caused by the menopause; the previous list represents some of the more common.

Symptoms as an Aid to Diagnosis

Understanding menopausal symptoms is important for two main reasons. First of all, they are significant tools in the diagnosis of menopause. Obviously, each woman only goes through the menopause once (thank goodness!) and therefore will not be able to draw upon past experience in order to understand the condition. At least when a woman reaches her premenstrual phase each month she knows, more or less, what will happen and why. Where the menopause is concerned, she not only has to deal with the fact that it is new territory, but she may find it very difficult to differentiate its symptoms from some of those that normally occur to her premenstrually.

As you will have recognized, some, if not many of the symptoms of the menopause are similar to those of PMT. Because there is no gap between menstrual years and menopausal onset it will be difficult to know for sure whether the menopause has begun or whether your menstrual cycle is just deviating from normal. As discussed earlier, there is a fairly wide variation in the average age for the menopause to set in. As a result, it is impossible for a woman just to assume that it is time for her to be starting the menopause. In this case the symptoms, along with a knowledge of the average menopausal age, may be of the utmost value in helping a woman to judge whether she is menopausal or not. Nevertheless, no diagnosis should be left completely to the individual; it should always be validated by a qualified health professional. Having said this, it is often women themselves who will alert their doctors that there is 'something amiss'.

Symptoms and Treatment Choice

The second reason it is important to understand the symptoms of the menopause is that this can aid you in your choice of treatment. Ordinarily when confronted with symptoms such as depression, headaches, fatigue, weight gain, etc. the inclination is to treat them with the usual remedies. However, when these symptoms are correlated with the menopause, 'normal' treatment may not be the best approach, for several reasons:

1. Symptomatic treatment of such symptoms may be less effective (or even ineffective) when directly or indirectly caused by hormonal imbalance.
2. Treatment of these symptoms may be unnecessary if the underlying cause (hormonal factors) is appropriately dealt with.
3. Some standard treatments for such symptoms may actually exacerbate the underlying hormonal difficulties which may have led to the symptoms in the first place.

For these reasons, as well as certain others, it is always best to know what your symptoms are being caused by, as it is always better to address the cause than just the symptoms. This does not only apply to the menopause; it applies to all health or medical problems. There may be times when certain symptoms will have to be treated individually, but at least if the cause has been determined, the most appropriate treatment (which is least likely to make the underlying problem worse) can be discovered and used.

Treating the cause of menopausal symptoms (which should help to relieve the symptoms as well) will be discussed in the next chapter. Treatments that will not negatively affect the underlying factors behind certain individual symptoms will also be covered.

CHAPTER 3

Causes of Menopausal Symptoms

When trying to treat menopausal difficulties it is extremely important to understand and deal with their underlying causes. This can seem a very confusing point for people, especially when they consider that the menopause itself is not a disorder *per se*.

Menopause is caused by a reduction and eventual cessation of menstrual periods, fertility and the ovarian production of oestrogen. Of course there is nothing out of the ordinary about this process, and therefore there is really no point in trying to prevent it from ever occurring. You may want to postpone the event as long as you can for obvious reasons, but it has to happen eventually. What this means is that the underlying causes can themselves only be dealt with up to a point.

When what should be a gradual and relatively uneventful transition becomes debilitating, disorderly and generally uncomfortable, that is the time to address it as a problem. The body is supposed to be able to adjust adequately to any changes. It is only when something negatively influences the parts of the body that control this transition that things become difficult.

THE GLANDS AND OESTROGEN

Pituitary and Hypothalamus

Perhaps the main area to consider is the role of the glands in the menopause. Up until the point of menopause, the ovaries are the primary site of oestrogen production. After this time, when the supply of egg-bearing follicles has been exhausted, the ovaries become unable to release oestrogen in response to the normal oestrogen-stimulating hormones. Logically, we might assume that the source of any menopausal difficulties would lie, therefore, in the pituitary or the hypothalamus; after all, it is these glands that are responsible for triggering the hormonal functioning of the ovaries in the first place. This may be true, but research has shown that the 'feedback' process which triggers the hormones relevant to the menstrual cycle appears to continue to function, at least to an extent, even after there is no longer an ability to produce oestrogen in the ovaries.

It is as though the pituitary and the hypothalamus are completely oblivious to what is happening in the ovaries during the menopause. This may be what leads some women to experience a difficult menopause. After all, the hypothalamus and the pituitary are certainly not immune from improper or erratic functioning; as a matter of fact they may be more susceptible due to the fact that they have more responsibilities than any other glands. If the ovaries can no longer produce oestrogen, yet the hormonal signals continue between the hypothalamus, the pituitary and the ovaries, it is not difficult to expect some biological confusion! While it is still unclear exactly how or why, the state of the hypothalamus and the pituitary glands prior to the menopause may determine, at least to an extent, how easy or difficult the menopausal transition can be.

Adrenal Glands

Perhaps the easiest glandular relationship to understand in menopause is that of the adrenals. This is also perhaps the most important relationship to consider when trying to make sense of the time leading up to the menopause and thereafter.

THE ADRENALS AND OESTROGEN

Throughout the menstrual years, the ovaries are not the only glands capable of manufacturing sex hormones. The adrenal glands, located on top of the kidneys, also manufacture oestrogen and androgens (male hormones). As mentioned earlier, the androgens are responsible for the sex drive in women (as well as in men).

The oestrogen manufactured by the adrenals is of particular value in both the transitional phase, as the menstrual years begin to wane, and in the years after the menopause occurs. In the run up to the menopause, there will still be some activity of ovarian oestrogen, albeit less than in previous years. At this time, the adrenal oestrogen will be a welcome complement to the reduced capability of the ovaries. However, after the follicles are exhausted and ovarian oestrogen stops, the adrenal oestrogen becomes the body's viable source. The adrenals will carry out this responsibility from then on. This sounds like a nice and tidy plan, and it is – provided everything is in proper working order.

BASIC FUNCTIONS

The adrenal glands have many responsibilities from the early stages of a woman's life. Among their many functions, they:

a) implement the body's response to stress
b) regulate inflammatory and allergic reactions
c) regulate blood sugar metabolism (along with the
   pancreas)
d) regulate sodium and potassium levels

Considering that the adrenal glands carry out so many essential processes, it is not difficult for them to become somewhat taxed by any undue strain. This is especially true in relation to their control of stress.

THE ADRENALS AND STRESS

Stress is a very general and ambiguous term, but it can basically be described as any factor that alters the body's 'status quo', or normal, intended function. This could mean emotional or mental stress, physical stress, environmental stress (such as temperature changes), etc. Of course, no one is immune from the wide variety of stressors in life.

The adrenal glands exert control in times of stress by releasing certain hormones such as *adrenaline*. Adrenaline is what accounts for the anxiety, nervousness and hyper-alertness which comes in the initial stages of stress. With long-term stress comes the release of *corticosteroids*, which are another class of adrenal hormones.

Stress can have a significant effect on the quality of a woman's experience of the menopause. One primary effect relates to the connection between stress and the common symptoms of the menopause.

ADRENALINE AND MENOPAUSAL SYMPTOMS

When a person is under stress for a short period, the release of hormones such as adrenaline produce the stimulating symptoms mentioned above. Unfortunately, no one is a 'bottomless pit' of adrenaline, therefore if the stress is chronic, there is the possibility that the supply and release of adrenaline may become inadequate and sluggish. This leads to fatigue, exhaustion, depression, etc. This may help to explain why at least some menopausal symptoms are significantly worse if a woman is regularly under stress. Of course, even the early symptoms of stress, such as anxiety and nervous tension, are also common symptoms of the menopause.

STRESS AND ADRENAL WEAKNESS

The second connection is related to the excessive demands put on the adrenal glands as a result of chronic stress. The more functions a particular part of the body is responsible for, the greater the likelihood that it will not be able to do all of them well. In other words, if a disproportionate amount of adrenal activity is having to go towards stabilizing the body under stress, then it may be less efficient at manufacturing and releasing ample amounts of sex hormones (e.g. oestrogen).

The implications of this are quite clear. As you know, the adrenal glands become the viable source of oestrogen in the body once the ovaries can no longer produce the hormone. If adrenal function is significantly weakened by chronic stress, oestrogen levels are bound to suffer – not to mention the fact that many of the symptoms of the menopause will be exacerbated by stress anyway.

For these reasons, it is very important to do whatever possible to avoid stress at this time (easier said than done!). Even if the stress cannot be avoided, as is generally the case, every effort must be made to strengthen and sustain the ability of the adrenal glands to function at a very high rate. Even if you are not under a great deal of stress during the menopausal stage, if chronic stress existed earlier in life, or if any other factor has weakened the adrenal glands, then steps must be taken to protect and strengthen these all-important glands. Methods of helping the adrenals to cope will be covered later.

Diet and Menopausal Symptoms

Diet is perhaps one of the most important factors to address when trying to prevent the menopause from being so debilitating. When we look at the factors which most influence the imbalances in the hypothalamus, pituitary and particularly the adrenal glands, dietary mismanagement may be at the top of the list. Now, dietary mismanagement does not only mean eating the types of foods that are 'bad for you'. It also refers to deficiencies in various nutrients that are known to maintain the proper function of the above glands, as well as of the entire reproductive system. This is a vast and detailed subject and will be discussed in greater depth in Chapters Seven and Eight.

Hysterectomy and Menopause

As you may already know, the cause of the menopause in many women is the surgical removal of the ovaries and uterus, also known as a *complete hysterectomy*. This is not to be confused with a partial hysterectomy, which usually refers to the removal of only the uterus (although sometimes one of the two ovaries will be removed).

The uterus is used to carry the growing fetus, but it is also involved in each menstrual cycle even when no fertilization has taken place. Of course, it is the shedding of the lining of the uterus that causes menstrual bleeding. The uterus is a prime target of the hormone progesterone, but the uterus can only be affected by this hormone if it has first been affected by oestrogen. The action of these two hormones on the uterus involves the thickening of the endometrium (uterine wall). The uterus would appear only to be 'of value' if a woman wanted to carry a baby. From a mechanical standpoint this may well be the case, but it is clear that it does play an indirect part in the functioning of the female sex hormones as well.

PARTIAL HYSTERECTOMY

The surgical removal of the uterus may be required due to the development of severe benign uterine growths or cysts or, in the worst cases, due to malignant tumours. Another common occurrence that often leads to partial hysterectomy is *endometriosis*, that is, the overgrowth of endometrial tissue. Although the uterus is an integral part of the menstrual cycle, a woman is far less likely to undergo severe negative effects after a hysterectomy if her ovaries are not removed as well.

COMPLETE HYSTERECTOMY

Major problems are likely to develop when a woman has received a complete hysterectomy, in other words, when her ovaries have been removed as well. Ovarian cancer or cysts are common reasons for this type of surgery. Some of the implications of this are obvious, as the ovaries represent the primary site of oestrogen production. Of course, the first priority of this surgery is that the source of the cysts or cancer is removed. The aftermath, though, can be quite distressing: a woman is plunged into an immediate state of menopause.

Many women who have had a complete hyster-ectomy are fairly young, at least by menopausal standards. If a woman receiving the surgery is, say, 35, then she is losing what would most likely have been 10 to 15 years of relatively normal reproductive function-ing. She also will take on the common symptoms of oestrogen loss far earlier than would otherwise have been the case.

Some feel that it is less debilitating to enter the menopause immediately than to do it gradually. However, it must be remembered that if the menopause approaches gradually, then the changes and/or symp-toms are more gradual as well. As a matter of fact, if the menopause develops in a proper manner, then the symptoms may be almost indiscernible in some women.

Once an early menopause has been produced by such surgery, the adrenal production of oestrogen becomes a major priority of the endocrine system. As has been discussed, a woman's reproductive system runs by a system of hormonal feedback (i.e. ovarian production occurs only if the hypothalamus and pituitary hormones tell it to begin). The same thing could be said for adrenal oestrogen. Even though the adrenals can produce some oestrogen during the menstrual years, when a woman moves towards menopause the pituitary signals the adrenals to produce more in order to compensate for the reduction in ovarian oestrogen. Who is to say that the pituitary can efficiently carry out these feedback tasks when the natural preparation process of a gradual menopause is removed? It is conceivable that interrupt-ing the intended 'winding down' process might reduce the adrenal glands' ability to adjust properly the output of oestrogen. The end result of this can be an extreme version of many of the common menopausal symptoms.

The point is, the human body is designed to function with all of its major parts intact. As a result, it is difficult to expect things to run normally when this is not the case.

If a hysterectomy is medically necessary then that should of course take priority. A woman should, however, be counselled on what to expect and what she can do afterwards so that she can prepare as best as possible. Again, a partial hysterectomy is far less likely to produce problems, but even if a woman has received a complete hysterectomy, there are methods (many both safe and natural) that may help relieve some or many of the symptoms that follow. These will be discussed in Chapters Six, Seven and Eight.

Menstruation and the Menopause

There is another problem that generally dictates just how difficult the menopausal transition will be. Even though the menopause has its own set of symptoms, for many women the adverse changes that accompany the transitional phase from menstruating to the menopause are even more bothersome.

The transitional phase represents the time period when the menstrual periods are drawing to a close. This 'phasing out' can occur in several different ways. There will be changes in the normal manner in which the periods occur, either in their frequency, their timing, the menstrual flow, or perhaps all of these. The nature of such changes will differ greatly from woman to woman. The following are some of the changes that might occur:

TRANSITIONAL CHANGES
• Menstrual periods may become gradually less

frequent than usual. The average menstrual period occurs approximately every 28 days. It is common, as the menopause approaches, for more and more time to elapse between periods, although this is not always the case

- The period and/or the various menstrual phases prior to the period may last for fewer or more days than would typically be the case. Although variable, in a 28-day cycle, menstruation lasts about four days, ovulation occurs on about day 14, and the premenstrual phase runs for the rest of the cycle until menstruation starts again

- The quantity of blood loss during menstruation may decrease or increase. It is thought that about 50 millilitres (ml) of blood is lost during an average menstrual phase. If significantly higher amounts are lost, this may (for a small proportion of women) signify a problem such as benign uterine cysts, endometriosis or, in rare instances, uterine cancer. Although such disorders are not typical, any woman who feels that there may be a cause for concern should have a checkup. If a woman experiences uterine bleeding *after* she has stopped having periods, she should alert her doctor immediately to rule out any major disorder such as the ones listed above

These menstrual changes listed above are those that are likely to occur as a woman moves toward the menopause. The changes are often quite gradual and thus produce little inconvenience; nevertheless it is not at all unusual for a woman to be greatly inconvenienced by them. Frequently there will be women who have such erratic and severe changes that they are unable even remotely to know what to expect.

Many women who experience very difficult premenstrual and menstrual disorders plan their lives around their cycles. This is understandable as some women are prone to severe emotional and physical dysfunction at varying stages of their cycle. If the timing or manifestation of the periods becomes unpredictable or erratic as menopause approaches, this can create a further source of stress.

PMT and the Menopause

Until fairly recently there was a gross misconception that premenstrual tension (PMT) was not a 'real' disorder. Fortunately, published medical and scientific research is changing this perception. The research, much of which was published in the *Journal of Reproductive Medicine* and *The Lancet*, has shown that PMT is primarily the result of hormonal imbalance.

A most useful finding in the studies showed that those women who were prone to high oestrogen and low progesterone levels during the premenstrual phase (approximately 70 per cent of those studied) tended toward irritability, mood swings and anxiety. The 25 to 30 per cent who were prone to high progesterone and low oestrogen, on the other hand, tended toward depression, memory lapse, crying spells and sleep disorders. It is also known that the hormones of the adrenal glands, the thyroid gland and the pituitary gland are in disarray in many cases of PMT.

About one out of every three women in her thirties suffers with PMT, so we can assume that hormonal imbalance of one sort or another is quite prevalent. With this in mind, imagine just how confusing the picture will be when such a woman gets close to the menopause.

It is this convoluted hormonal picture that makes the pre-menopausal period so unpredictable and disconcerting. Because it is during the menstrual periods of this transitional time that some of the most distressing symptoms can occur, it is important to understand, in basic terms, the truth behind PMT.

It seems almost assured that a woman who has terrible PMT prior to the menopause is more likely to have a terrible time in the menopause. The main reason for this is quite simple. Since PMT is caused by a disorder and imbalance of certain glands (the pituitary, hypothalamus, adrenals, etc.), there is no reason to expect this problem to get any better as a woman gets older. If anything, we can assume that in many cases it would get worse, unless there were some positive and significant changes made in overall health, diet, or perhaps stress levels.

PMT SUBGROUPS

There are four basic classes of PMT. Each class represents a different hormonal pattern and manifests a different set of symptoms. It may seem confusing, but knowing the particular subgroup you fit into can help in the diagnosis and treatment of PMT and is particularly important as you approach menopause.

Subclasses of PMT

PMT-A

Common symptoms include:

- irritability and tension
- anxiety
- mood swings

In this type of PMT a woman is prone to elevated levels of oestrogen and lower levels of progesterone. Between two-thirds to three-quarters of all sufferers fall into this subclass.

PMT-C
Common symptoms include:
- tendency towards cravings
- appetite increases
- dizziness
- tiredness
- headaches
- heart palpitations

Blood sugar imbalances appear to be a significant factor in this type of PMT. The research has also found that deficiencies in a hormone-like substance called *prostaglandin E1* may be involved in some cases. Such a deficiency may increase the risk of this blood sugar abnormality. This type may affect one-quarter to one-third of PMT sufferers.

PMT-D
Common symptoms include:
- depression
- sleep disorders
- crying spells
- memory lapse

This type of PMT, which is about as prevalent as PMT-C, is correlated with elevated progesterone and low oestrogen levels. It would appear to be a total opposite of PMT-A, however it must be remembered that the hormone levels can fluctuate greatly during the course of the premenstrual phase. After all, there are many women who experience both anxiety and depression during the same cycle.

PMT-H

Common symptoms include:

- weight gain
- retention of fluid
- bloating
- breast pain and/or tenderness

PMT-H is a very common form affecting about 70 per cent of all PMT sufferers. Women in this category are prone to add more than three lb of weight premenstrually. It would appear that this weight increase (as well as the other PMT-H symptoms) is primarily being caused by an adrenal hormone called *aldosterone*, which causes the body to retain fluid.

These subclasses of PMT can help to explain what is probably going on hormonally, but it is clear that a woman can fall into more than one subclass. It is not a bad idea for any woman approaching the menopause to record her common and most severe symptoms and try to fit them into these subclasses. If a woman can succeed in reducing some of the hormonal factors that cause her to suffer with pre-menopausal PMT, she may well reduce the severity of her impending menopausal symptoms (see Chapters Six and Seven).

CHAPTER 4

Osteoporosis

Perhaps the most disturbing possible aspect of the menopause is *osteoporosis*. The condition has been gaining much publicity over the last decade or so and this, in turn, has raised the profile of the menopause in general. This is a fortunate development in that it has prompted much needed scientific and medical research into the causes and appropriate treatments of osteoporosis.

WHAT IS OSTEOPOROSIS?

Osteoporosis is a condition in which the bones become porous and weak. Osteoporosis has often been confused with another condition called *osteomalacia*. Osteomalacia refers to soft bones caused only by a lack of the mineral *calcium*. When most people think of osteoporosis, they often think that it, too, is caused by a lack of calcium, as this has been the 'watch word' of much of the publicity and education surrounding osteoporosis. The truth is that human bone tissue is made up of many different constituents. The mineral calcium is the single most plentiful mineral of the bones, but they also need several other minerals, as well as non-mineral constituents, in order to be healthy.

The main minerals needed in bone tissue include, among others, calcium, *phosphorus, magnesium, silicon* and *zinc*. If any of these or if any of the other minerals involved in the bones is deficient, then the result will be a weakening of the bone.

The non-mineral substances in the bone do not get much publicity at all. This is quite unfortunate because they are just as necessary as the minerals for healthy bone tissue. These constituents actually form what is sometimes known as the *matrix* of the bone. This matrix serves, more or less, as a cement to bind the mineral base together. Perhaps a good analogy of their function is to imagine a house built with bricks – but no mortar. It just wouldn't work, would it? Well, if you had plenty of calcium and other minerals, but were lacking ample 'bone mortar', then your bones would not hold together.

The substances that make up this non-mineral matrix are primarily proteins such as *collagen*. Collagen is the most abundant protein in the body and is a major component of all of your body's connective tissue, such as that in the skin, bones, blood vessels, etc. In order to promote proper bone health and integrity, all efforts must be made not only to ensure an adequate dietary intake of minerals, but also of matrix materials.

Osteoporosis involves damage to both the mineral and the non-mineral portion of the bone. Women are actually about four times more likely to develop osteoporosis than men.

Symptoms
Those who develop osteoporosis are likely to suffer symptoms such as:

- high susceptibility to fractures
- loss of height
- pain in the most affected areas

Osteoporosis symptoms are very different from those of other conditions in the way that they develop. In many other disorders, symptoms usually represent an early warning sign. In osteoporosis, it appears that discernible symptoms may not occur until a significant amount (about 30 per cent) of bone density has already been lost.

SPONTANEOUS FRACTURES

Often we think of the effects of osteoporosis only when we hear a story of some elderly woman who falls and breaks her hip. However, what often occurs is that the person's hip breaks first, which causes her to fall. This is what is known as a *spontaneous fracture*, and it is one of the most dreaded aspects of osteoporosis.

LOSS OF HEIGHT

The loss of height caused by osteoporosis is primarily due to the degeneration of the spinal column. What can also occur, however, is a severe curvature or hump in the back caused by the deformity of the affected bones. We associate this with the very old, but this is not always the case.

The hips and spine, as well as the ribs and knees, appear to be affected by osteoporosis much more than other areas. Particularly in the case of the hips, spine and knees, the fact that they are 'weight-bearing' joints makes them so susceptible to degeneration. The more weight being supported by a particular part of the body, the more stress and damage are bound to occur. The more damage caused to bones, the more the body is called upon to repair them. If this reparation is not forthcoming due to an inadequate supply of bone materials, then the area may weaken to the point at which the bones can no longer support the necessary weight. This causes the loss of height and/or a higher likelihood of fractures.

You do not have to be in your seventies or eighties to suffer the consequences of osteoporosis, although the older you get the more likely you are to have problems of this sort. It is also important to note that osteoporosis does not happen overnight. It generally takes many years to develop, but it does so quietly and, as mentioned, often without any noticeable symptoms for quite some time. In women the bones may start to lose their density quite early on, while they are still in their thirties, although it is thought that the first major signs may occur around the age of 40. A moderate loss of bone mass is not really abnormal and does not mean a woman will develop osteoporosis. However, once a woman reaches menopausal age the rate of bone loss may speed up considerably. The vast majority of women past the menopausal age will experience considerable bone loss.

Causes
There are many reasons why osteoporosis may develop. As mentioned, the body needs a supply of several different substances in order to manufacture healthy bone. Many of the substances that are required, such as calcium, magnesium, phosphorus, zinc, etc. are classified as *essential nutrients*.

DIET AND NUTRIENTS
An essential nutrient is a nutrient that is required in order to live but which cannot be made in the body in adequate amounts; therefore they must be supplied in the diet. If you are deficient in any of the essential

nutrients involved in bone building, then there will be problems. As a result, what you eat can play a huge role in combating the risk of developing osteoporosis.

Although the non-mineral proteins in the bone matrix (collagen, osteocalcin, etc.) are not essential nutrients, they cannot be made unless certain essential nutrients are present in the body in adequate amounts.

Some nutrients are not actually constituents of bones, but are needed none the less in order for the bone tissue to be replenished. Vitamin D is an example of such a nutrient. A deficiency in vitamin D has disastrous effects on bone density. The bottom line is that diet cannot be disregarded no matter what is causing the osteoporosis. The effect of diet on osteoporosis will be covered in detail in Chapters Six and Seven.

LACK OF EXERCISE

Lack of exercise is another problem for bone strength. When a woman exercises, she puts a certain amount of stress on her frame. While severe stress can damage the skeleton, the moderate stress from sensible exercise actually stimulates the frame to repair itself even though no significant damage has taken place.

MEDICATION

Certain drugs have also been implicated in premature bone loss. *Corticosteroids* are among the most destructive to the bones. These are sometimes given to treat inflammatory, allergic or auto-immune disorders such as rheumatoid arthritis. Other medications can produce a problem as well, but corticosteroids are among the worst culprits.

ALCOHOL, CAFFEINE, NICOTINE AND SUGAR

Alcohol, caffeine, nicotine and sugar represent serious threats to the integrity of the bones. Because of the sheer volume and frequency in which these substances are often consumed, one or all of them must be considered as the major factors in some cases of osteoporosis. For more details see Chapter Six.

MENOPAUSE AND OSTEOPOROSIS

We generally think of bone as a static substance. Nothing could be further from the truth. The bone tissue in your body is constantly being broken down and then regenerated. This is a natural and necessary process.

Hormones and Bone Tissue

Bone tissue is broken down by cells called *osteoclasts*. Bone tissue is built up by cells called *osteoblasts*. These cells carry out the chemical commands of certain hormones. Osteoclasts are controlled by the action of *parathyroid hormone* from the parathyroid glands found in the thyroid gland. Osteoblasts are controlled by a hormone called *calcitonin*.

The main hormone involved in bone density is *1,25 dihydroxy-cholecalciferol*. It would be much easier to refer to this hormone by its initial form, *vitamin D*. 1,25 dihydroxy-cholecalciferol is made from vitamin D in the kidneys after a fairly complicated process. The main role of vitamin D in bone building is that it is needed for the absorption of calcium. This will be expanded on later.

Parathyroid hormone, besides breaking down bone, ironically increases calcium absorption and retention in the body. It also helps the conversion of vitamin D into its most active form.

Calcitonin, by helping bone to be rebuilt, actually lowers calcium levels in the blood, which then triggers parathyroid hormone, and so on. This process goes back and forth in a cycle, one hormone triggering the other and the end result hopefully being a maintenance of bone strength and fresh healthy tissue. Now you can begin to see the delicate balance in the way the body maintains its skeletal structure. Unfortunately, it would appear that this process begins to lose its underpinnings somewhat during the menopause.

Oestrogen Loss and Osteoporosis

It is thought that when oestrogen levels fall during the menopause, osteoclasts increase the rate of bone breakdown in response to parathyroid hormone. This breakdown of bone causes the bone calcium to flood the bloodstream. This process signals a *decrease* in the output of parathyroid hormone. This in turn reduces both the absorption and retention of calcium, which leads to bone weakening. (Remember, besides breaking down bone, parathyroid hormone also increases calcium absorption in the intestines and calcium retention.)

The end result of the increased sensitivity of the osteoclasts to parathyroid hormone is that the normal cycle is interrupted and only the phase during which bone is broken down seems to continue. The part of the cycle in which the absorption and retention of calcium is increased seems to be impeded.

This theory, though complex and perhaps confusing, would explain one reason for the increased speed in the breakdown of bone associated with the menopause. There are other reasons, which will be covered in Chapter Six.

CHAPTER 5

Medical Treatment
of Menopausal Symptoms

One of the most controversial issues surrounding the menopause concerns its treatment. Every woman deserves better than to suffer throughout the menopausal transition with debilitating symptoms; in order for many women to avoid this, some form of treatment may have to be utilized. Many women who seek help for their menopausal symptoms, especially those who are found to have a high risk of osteoporosis, will probably be made aware of hormone replacement treatment (HRT).

HRT

HRT involves a medical replacement of oestrogen. At this time the most common forms include pills, cremes, patches and implants (see chart below). Each form has its own practical advantages over the others, depending on the needs of each woman.

Possible Benefits of HRT

The premise behind HRT seems, on the surface, to be sensible in that if a woman's symptoms are caused by an oestrogen deficiency, then replacing the oestrogen should relieve the symptoms. This is where part of the controversy arises, however. Nevertheless, research appears to confirm that HRT can be of value in relieving *some* of the symptoms in many women, including:

- Hot flushes/night sweats.
- Vaginal disorders. Vaginal cremes are often used locally in order to avoid as many of the systemic (throughout the body) effects of the oestrogen. This may help restore vaginal integrity and thus reduce or eliminate pain during intercourse.
- Osteoporosis. (Please note that using HRT does *not* eliminate the need for ensuring that all the necessary constituents of bone are being supplied in the diet!)
- Heart attack and strokes. Oestrogen may reduce a tendency for excessive clotting of the blood, which can be associated with the menopause. Ironically, there is also thought to be a slightly *increased* risk of heart attack and stroke in certain women who use HRT. This would be the case particularly if progestogens had to be used along with the oestrogen.

Emotional Symptoms and HRT
It seems that the track record of HRT in other menopausal symptoms, such as those that involve emotional changes, is not very good. Although some women may receive benefits in such cases, no one should automatically expect to feel better in terms of mood, emotional instability or depression when on HRT. As a matter of fact, mood swings are one of the more common side-effects of HRT in some women.

Risks and Side-effects Associated with HRT
It is important to be aware of the side-effects associated with HRT. They do not always outweigh the benefits but, as with all medical treatments, they should be

understood if you are considering the treatment. Some of the more well-documented risks of HRT include:

- Uterine cancer. As oestrogen causes the uterine lining to thicken, if this hormone alone is being given continually it can cause the lining to overgrow in some cases. This can increase the risk of cancer of the womb. Such occurrences are relatively rare due to the fact that such hormones are often balanced with progestogens, which cause the lining of the womb to shed. The risks are highest in long-term use, especially at higher doses. This risk would not exist in those women who had received a hysterectomy prior to starting HRT.
- Breast cancer. Although the risk is relatively low, women with a history or higher risk of breast cancer should avoid HRT. Those with fibrocystic breast disease or a family history of breast cancer should alert their doctor of such a history before using HRT.
- Weight gain/fluid retention. It is common for a woman to gain weight in fluid after beginning HRT.
- Mood swings.
- Depression.
- Headaches.
- Increased blood pressure.
- Gall stones.

The use of HRT affects one woman very differently from another. You should definitely weigh the benefits and the risks and should encourage your doctor to discuss such implications openly.

Complete Hysterectomy and HRT

One particularly grey area is in the case of complete hysterectomy. If a woman has had her ovaries removed at a comparatively early age (such as in her mid-thirties), she is probably many years away from the time when she would have started the menopause naturally. The loss of oestrogen, as well as the impending symptoms and osteoporosis that might develop were HRT not to be used, make it difficult to disagree with the use of HRT provided all of the risks have been addressed and/or are monitored. The surgical removal of the ovaries is not a natural process and may therefore have to be treated in an 'unnatural' way; for this reason many of those who are ordinarily against the use of HRT may actually support it in such a case.

Weighing the Options

Whether or not to use HRT is a very personal decision which should only be taken after consultation with a specialist, with all the relevant information, positive and negative, being discussed.

PLEASE NOTE: If the decision has been made to use HRT, *never* discontinue use without first consulting your doctor. Immediate or unmonitored stoppage of HRT can result in a worsening of symptoms in some women.

Some Common Hormone Replacement Drugs

HRT TREATMENT	MADE WITH
Pills:	
conjugated oestrogens	*natural oestrogens*
mestranol	*semi-synthetic oestrogen*
norethisterone	*progestogen*
Patches:	
oestradiol	*natural oestrogen*
Vaginal Cremes:	
oestriol	*natural oestrogen*
conjugated oestrogens	*natural oestrogen*
dienoestrol	*natural oestrogen*

CHAPTER 6

Diet and the Treatment of Menopausal Symptoms and Osteoporosis

There is no question that the menopause is potentially one of the most difficult times in life for many women. Even though not all women will have a terrible time, most would still like to combat even the minor symptoms of the menopause. Also, whether experiencing symptoms or not, fears about osteoporosis have prompted many women to seek preventative treatment. The problem is, there is so much conflicting information that many will end up more confused than before about the best approach to take.

THE GROWING EMPHASIS ON NATURAL APPROACH

The controversies relating to the replacement of oestrogen in the menopause have concerned many women seeking treatment for their symptoms. This has prompted many to look elsewhere, particularly into natural methods of relieving the symptoms or reducing the risks of osteoporosis. This area, while free from the levels of risk or side-effects associated with HRT, can be very confusing as well, particularly because there are so many alternatives.

The medical community often sends rather mixed signals as to the value of such alternatives – in general, this is probably due to a lack of awareness of the proven value of various non-drug therapies. This trend is clearly changing, however, as the overwhelming volume of evidence supporting natural medicine becomes more heavily publicized.

This chapter and Chapter Seven (as well as Chapter Five) are dedicated to setting the record straight. In order to avoid as much confusion as possible, all of the information on natural treatments is based primarily on published medical and scientific research. Fortunately there is a large amount of scientific evidence supporting the positive benefits to be gained by changing your diet, as well as by using nutrient and herbal therapies in the treatment of menopausal disorders. This chapter will focus on diet.

THE EARLY INFLUENCE OF DIET

Menopause itself may begin for most women in their mid-forties to early fifties, but the factors that determine whether the menopause will be difficult or easy surface long before then. As mentioned earlier, in many cases the tendency toward imbalances in glandular activity related to reproductive functioning may be evident during the menstrual years. This is not guaranteed, but if you have suffered from some glandular problems and no major change occurs in your physiology or biochemistry, it is unlikely that these problems will spontaneously disappear.

If such problems occur consistently, they will probably have a great deal to do with certain aspects of a woman's diet and lifestyle, perhaps even more than with some genetic or congenital glandular abnormality. As a matter of fact, research has proven that there is a significant and direct link between dietary intake and PMT.

Dietary Excesses and PMT

As far as excessive intake of foods is concerned, research published in the *Journal of Reproductive Medicine* in 1983 confirmed that PMT sufferers consumed more than 75 per cent more dairy products and sodium than those who did not suffer with PMT. Even more shocking was the statistic that showed that PMT sufferers consumed nearly 300 per cent more refined sugar than women who did not suffer from PMT! Just a coincidence?

Deficiencies and PMT

There is ample evidence to suggest the way in which such excesses would account for glandular, and thus hormonal, disturbances. Research has also shown that female hormonal difficulties were linked not only to dietary excesses but to a significantly lower intake of certain essential nutrients compared with that of non-sufferers. Some of these nutrients included the minerals zinc and iron and the vitamins B_6 and pantothenic acid (B_5).

It is clear that female hormonal problems, and thus their correction, depend not only on what you put into your body but also on what you do *not* put into it. Getting the balance right may have unimaginable benefits for your hormonal state of health.

Examples of dietary mismanagement, such as those listed above, are not restricted to PMT sufferers. Examples exist in menopausal women as well. As you will find in Part 1 of this chapter, the implications of such factors can be quite damaging.

NEGATIVE FOODS

There are several substances that can be detrimental to proper hormonal functioning. Either they may reduce the activity of certain hormones or, conversely, they may cause excessive hormonal activity. Several foods can also have an adverse effect on certain symptoms as well as on bone density, regardless of any effect on specific hormones.

Alcohol

Some of the worst substances are not actually foods at all. Alcohol is a perfect example. In the case of PMT studies, levels of the vitamins B_1, B_2, B_6 and niacin and of the mineral zinc and others have been found to be very much lower in PMT sufferers than in non-sufferers. As it turns out, alcohol can adversely affect either the absorption or utilization of, or cause the depletion of all of these nutrients.

BONE NUTRIENTS AND ALCOHOL

Other nutrients that are negatively affected include magnesium and calcium. Magnesium has been proven to be incredibly effective at reducing many symptoms of the premenstrual phase, including fluid-related weight gain, breast tenderness and nervous tension. Calcium especially but also magnesium and zinc are absolutely essential in order to maintain proper bone strength and density. A deficiency in these, as well as in other nutrients that are negatively affected by alcohol, would lead to an increased risk of osteoporosis.

FATTY ACID DISTURBANCE

Another damaging effect of alcohol is on the conversion

of what are known as *dietary fatty acids*. Dietary fatty acids are derived from fats in the food you eat. One of the types alcohol interferes with is the fatty acid that has been found to correct certain female hormonal disorders. This is called *cis-linoleic acid*.

ALCOHOL AND LIVER FUNCTION

Perhaps the most well-known adverse effect of alcohol is on the liver. The reduction in liver functioning is particularly pertinent in female hormonal problems due to the fact that the liver processes and detoxifies such hormones. The ability of the liver to break down hormonal components is essential to protect the body from certain toxic effects that these hormones may have. The inability of this breakdown to occur efficiently appears to be linked to many of the side-effects of the contraceptive pill, such as headaches and the increased risk of breast and uterine disorders. The same would be true of HRT. For this reason, alcohol should especially be avoided when a woman is receiving hormonal therapy with oestrogens.

ALCOHOL AND STRESS

We have already covered some of the adverse effects of stress on the menopause. The primary problem is related to the weakening of the functioning of the adrenal glands in general, which may occur if the stress is chronic. This is particularly important because, as mentioned earlier, the adrenal glands become the only source of oestrogen once the ovaries cease production after the menopause.

Stress is not the only factor that causes a stimulation and over-taxing of the adrenal glands. Alcohol also causes this to occur. After alcohol is consumed there is a rise in the release of adrenaline. Adrenaline has many effects on the body that would exacerbate menopausal problems:

- adrenaline can cause anxiety, tension, and irritability.
- adrenaline constricts the blood vessels (vasoconstriction). As hot flushes and night sweats are caused by a circulatory defect in which the blood vessels release blood flow erratically, menopausal woman should avoid anything that further adversely affects circulation.
- adrenaline raises the blood pressure. Women who are put on HRT may have an increased risk of high blood pressure anyway, so adrenaline-increasing agents should be avoided.

ADRENAL EXHAUSTION

As you may recall, no one has an unending supply of adrenaline; the hormone must be manufactured constantly. If this is not done efficiently, our tolerance for stress is reduced. This can lead to a significant worsening of the emotional as well as some of the physical symptoms of the menopause.

It is also important to remember that if the adrenal glands are working too hard (because of excessive stress or the consumption of adrenaline stimulating agents such as alcohol), 'adrenal exhaustion' can easily occur. This would lead not only to low stress tolerance but also fatigue, depression and many other negative symptoms.

Smoking

There is no lack of information on the negative effects of smoking on health. Looking more deeply into the specific effects of both tars and nicotine shows that smoking is likely to be particularly destructive to menopausal women.

SMOKING AND OSTEOPOROSIS

Smoking drains certain important nutrients from your body very quickly, especially *vitamin C*. Vitamin C, also known as ascorbic acid, has several essential purposes in the body. Perhaps the best known is its strengthening effect on the immune system. Particularly relevant to the menopause is the fact that vitamin C is the primary nutrient needed in order to build collagen. As collagen is the chief substance involved in the non-mineral matrix of the bone, any inadequacy of vitamin C levels would lead to a deficiency in collagen, and thus a far greater risk of osteoporosis.

SMOKING AND THE ADRENAL GLANDS

Alcohol is certainly not the only substance that causes a release of adrenaline from the adrenal glands. The active stimulant in tobacco is *nicotine*. Nicotine causes a significant release of adrenaline. This accounts to a great extent for the rush of alertness and mental energy received from smoking. Unfortunately, this also accounts for the increased tendencies for high blood pressure, nervous tension and irritability associated with tobacco.

The rush of adrenaline caused by nicotine makes the blood vessels constrict. As a result, smoking may exacerbate the circulatory problems (hot flushes and night sweats) associated with the menopause.

As with alcohol, the over-stimulation of the adrenal glands caused by smoking can weaken these glands, perhaps reducing their ability to manufacture oestrogen as efficiently as is required during the menopause.

CIGARETTE SMOKE AND REPRODUCTIVE CANCERS

The actual smoke from cigarettes affects more than just the lungs. Among other things, the smoke contains harmful substances called *free radicals* as well as dangerous heavy metals. Free radicals can cause healthy cells in the body to mutate. When such cells multiply in a mutated form, then cancer can be formed. Although such problems primarily affect the respiratory tract, certain harmful agents may affect other tissues as well, including those in the reproductive area.

Caffeine

Another class of drugs that are regularly consumed drugs is from the family called *methylxanthine*, of which caffeine is a member. Caffeine and its related chemicals are found in coffee, tea, chocolate, many soft drinks and some pain relievers. Caffeine is one of the most popular stimulants and is readily available and legal for people of all ages. As a result, many have come to the erroneous conclusion that it is safe and free of any major side-effects over the long term. While most people are aware that if you drink too much coffee, for instance, you may have difficulty sleeping or become nervous, these are just caffeine's more minor side-effects.

CAFFEINE AND THE ADRENALS

Caffeine is yet another example of a drug that causes the release of excessive amounts of adrenaline. Many of the short-term (as well as long-term) side-effects of caffeine consumption are caused by caffeine-induced adrenaline. These include irritability, nervous tension, insomnia, high blood pressure, etc. The direct effects of adrenaline listed under alcohol and nicotine would also apply to caffeine, including adrenal weakness and circulatory problems.

COFFEE, TEA AND NUTRITIONAL DEFICIENCIES

Coffee and tea pose some major concerns for meno-pausal women besides just their effect on the adrenals. Both zinc and iron are victims of these beverages in that they reduce the body's ability to absorb these minerals. This can easily lead to iron deficiency anaemia, as well as to an increased risk of osteoporosis as a result of a zinc deficiency. Caffeine is a diuretic as well – that is, it causes rapid fluid elimination which can cause the loss of important hormonal and bone-enhancing nutrients as well. Research has shown that there is a substantial loss of calcium in the urine after caffeine ingestion. Caffeine may also interfere with the beneficial effect of oestrogen on calcium utilization.

CAFFEINE AND BREAST PROBLEMS

Research has found that caffeine consumption is one of the major causes of breast tenderness and pain pre-menstrually, as well as of fibrocystic breast lumps or cysts. In associated research, almost all of the women who eliminated the methylxanthines (caffeine, theo-phylline, theobromine) found in tea, coffee, etc. had a reduction in their fibrocystic breast symptoms.

Sugar

Many people will be aware of some of the damaging effects of the substances named so far, but very few people take sugar quite so seriously. Sugar poses an interesting dichotomy. It represents a major source of fuel to keep our bodies running, but at the same time it can cause untold damage if too much is consumed and/or if it is consumed in an improper form.

SIMPLE VERSUS COMPLEX CARBOHYDRATES

The body needs sugar to live, but sugar in excess of what the body requires for its immediate energy needs can cause problems.

Foods that contain sugars can be consumed in one of two basic forms – *simple carbohydrates* or *complex carbohydrates*.

Some examples of simple carbohydrates include:

- white and brown sugar
- honey
- fruits and juices
- fructose
- glucose
- dextrose

A simple carbohydrate contains sugar in a more readily usable form. If a person consumes sugar as a simple carbohydrate then the bloodstream receives the sugar more quickly. Depending on the amounts consumed, this may well be much more than the body can metabolize to use for energy. If this occurs, the excess sugar may be stored, at least to an extent, as fat. On the other hand, excessive insulin release after sugar intake may, ironically, lead to 'rebound' hypoglycaemia (low blood sugar). This can cause weakness, exhaustion, depression and other related symptoms.

Although fresh fruits are a source of simple carbohydrates, they are less likely to pose such problems as their fibre and water content reduce the concentration of sugar that enters the bloodstream.

Complex carbohydrates are a source of sugar as well, but in this case they come in the form of *starches*. Common sources of complex carbohydrates include:

- *whole* grains (brown rice, whole wheat, oats, barley, rye, etc.)
- potatoes
- beans/legumes

These carbohydrates are called complex because the sugars they contain are bonded with fibre. This bonding causes the sugar to be released much more gradually than is the case with simple carbohydrates. This leads to more stable levels of blood sugar and avoids the side-effects associated with excess sugar consumption. Also, complex carbohydrate foods generally contain much higher levels of vitamins and minerals, which are needed in order to use the sugars properly in the first place.

SUGAR AND ADRENAL FUNCTION
The consumption of refined sugar (sucrose, glucose, etc.) is linked to adrenaline release. You are already well aware of what damage this can do and the fact that sugar is a stimulant tends to add to its addictive properties.

SUGAR AND OSTEOPOROSIS
Calcium is lost in the urine in larger quantities after the consumption of sugar. Because of this, excessive intake of sugar should be avoided in order to maintain bone density.

SUGAR AND BREAST CANCER
Medical research has shown a definite connection between the intake of sugar and an increased risk of breast cancer. This link appears to be especially valid in women over 45 years old. While it is still unclear as to the exact reason for the increased risk, two factors have been suggested:

1. A low-fibre diet has been shown to reduce the speedy elimination of certain cancer-causing agents. High sugar diets have been found to be generally low in fibre.
2. Large amounts of sugar can significantly reduce the activity of certain immune cells known to destroy cancer cells.

There is another link between alcohol, caffeine, nicotine and sugar: If a person reduces the intake of one or more of this group, whether voluntarily or not, he or she is likely to increase the intake of another in the group to compensate. Because many of the negative effects of these substances on the menopause are fairly similar, trading one for another may not be very helpful. If you are trying to cut down on using one of these substances, do not increase your intake of another. The best plan is to eliminate or significantly reduce all of them, gradually, from your life. Succeeding in doing so may reduce the tendency toward menopausal problems such as low adrenal oestrogen output, hot flushes, emotional and mental difficulties, and so on. It also may reduce the risk of osteoporosis. Eliminating these substances may also cut down on premenstrual symptoms if you have not yet reached the menopause.

Excessive Protein and Osteoporosis
The adverse effect an ill-conceived diet can have on the menopause is substantial. One of the best examples of this actually has no direct correlation with reproductive hormones at all, and involves the development of osteoporosis.

One of the main contributors to a risk of osteoporosis is a diet that is high in protein. This may seem to contradict the received wisdom that protein is necessary for health. Nevertheless, a high-protein diet has been proved to be linked to an increased loss of calcium in the urine. This appears to be due to the fact that when high amounts of protein are consumed, this speeds up the filtering of certain substances (including calcium) from the blood into the urinary tract to be excreted. Another effect is that high amounts of protein reduce the rate of re-absorption of calcium in the part of the urinary tract called the renal tubes. The end result is lower calcium levels and thus weaker bones.

Some of the higher protein foods include:

- meat
- poultry
- fish
- eggs
- dairy products
- beans

Vegetarians, Meat Eaters and Osteoporosis

Studies have shown that those women who follow a vegetarian diet lose less bone density over a period of time than do meat-eaters. There are several possible explanations for this:

1. Vegetarian diets often contain a smaller concentration of protein than the diets of meat-eaters.
   This, of course, is not always the case, as milk products and eggs are very high in protein. However, the next two possibilities may explain the higher bone density that exist in vegetarians.
2. Most vegetarian diets are likely to contain less of the mineral phosphorus in proportion to calcium.

3. Most vegetarian diets are likely to contain far more calcium and other bone nutrients than do most meat-eaters' diets.

Phosphorus and Osteoporosis

As mentioned earlier, the bones are not static tissue. They are constantly being broken down and replaced. Parathyroid hormone, which is stimulated by phosphorus intake, is the hormone that causes the bones to be broken down. Calcitonin, which is stimulated by calcium intake, is the hormone that causes the bones to be rebuilt. Together these two hormones control the 'back and forth' process of maintaining bone.

If the blood levels of calcium are too low to maintain the other parts of the body that need calcium, calcium will be released from the bone to top up the blood levels. It may not seem that reducing your intake of phosphorus in relation to that of calcium would actually benefit bone strength, but if the balance between the levels of these two minerals shifts so that there is too much phosphorus, bone breakdown will exceed the rate of bone rebuilding, with the end result being bone loss. If the levels of phosphorus are far in excess of the required levels for a long period of time, this may lead to osteoporosis. As a result, for healthy bones the balance between calcium and phosphorus must be right.

In the *Journal of Nutrition* in 1977, a study was published that stated that there was significant bone loss in monkeys who consumed a ratio of about 2 to 1 phosphorus to calcium. When the ratio was changed to 1 to 1, there was no appreciable bone loss. Presumably, this would more or less hold true for humans. Unfortunately, it is thought that the 2 to 1 phosphorus-to-calcium ratio (or even worse) is what can be found in the typical Western diet! So just what makes the typical 'Western diet' so damaging to the bones?

Phosphorus, like calcium, is an essential nutrient that cannot be made by the body and must be supplied by the diet. While sources of calcium are less plentiful than you might think (*see page 84*), phosphorus is almost too plentiful in the typical Western diet. And while many food sources (such as dairy products and vegetables) are rich in phosphorus as well as being fairly rich in calcium, there is one major food that does not fall into this category: meat.

Meat, and particularly red meat, contains huge amounts of phosphorus and very little calcium. It would appear that the ratio of phosphorus to calcium in red meat is in the vicinity of between 20 and 30 to 1! It doesn't take much to imagine the net effect of this huge imbalance over a period of years. Therefore, if a menopausal woman has been eating meat (especially red meat) perhaps a few times a week for many years, it is no wonder that osteoporosis is such a risk.

SOFT DRINKS AND OSTEOPOROSIS

'Junk' foods and beverages have also played their role in the ever-decreasing standard of health in Western societies. Soft drinks such as colas are a prime example. Besides the fact that most have large amounts of sugar and many contain caffeine (both of which cause calcium loss), many varieties also contain phosphoric acid. As its name implies, this acid is connected with phosphorus. It is used in soft drinks to 'buffer' their acidity, which could otherwise cause tooth decay.

Negative Fats and the Menopause

Dietary fats come in many forms. Some are beneficial to

health, others may be detrimental. The main forms of dietary fats are polyunsaturated fats, saturated fats, and cholesterol. There are many different ways in which the wrong type of fats can affect health. They are too numerous to go into here, but one of the major parts of the body that can be adversely influenced is the circulatory system.

SATURATED FATS AND CHOLESTEROL

Saturated fats are primarily the fats that become solid at room temperature. Cholesterol is a blood fat that is used to make various hormones. The main sources of these include meats, dairy products and eggs. Saturated fat intake and high blood cholesterol levels are strongly implicated in heart disease. One main reason is that they can steadily impede circulation by causing the blood to clot excessively.

Menopausal women have an increased risk of heart disease anyway, due to the decreased level of oestrogen in their bodies. Anything that could exacerbate such a tendency, including excessive consumption of saturated fats, should be avoided. Circulatory defects also play a part in the propensity for hot flushes and night sweats. For this reason it may also be helpful to avoid saturated fats and keep blood cholesterol levels under control.

Animal fats in general have also been associated with an increased risk of breast cancer. If HRT is being used (which in itself carries a risk of breast cancer, especially in women with a family history of the disease), it may be advisable to reduce any other risk factors, including the intake of sources of food high in animal fats such as red meat and dairy products.

OXIDIZED POLYUNSATURATED FATS

Polyunsaturated fats (found in vegetables, seeds, nuts, grains, etc.) are considered by many to be the 'good' or 'healthy' form of fat and are indeed the dietary source of *essential fatty acids* (EFAs). As with essential vitamins or minerals, essential fatty acids are needed in order for us to live but must be supplied by the diet. Polyunsaturated fats are not free of controversy, however. All of the good things about them apply *only* if they are not damaged by either excessive heat, processing, or exposure to oxygen.

Cooking polyunsaturated fats damages their goodness (causing oxidation) and can make them potentially quite harmful. In this oxidized form they actually increase the risk of heart disease and excessive blood clotting; they increase the tendency toward inflammatory conditions (such as arthritis), and they may increase the risk of certain forms of cancer. This is due to the fact that oxidation produces free radicals, which can cause abnormal cells to develop.

A menopausal woman may feel free to consume polyunsaturated fats provided they are fresh and have not been used in cooking (especially frying). Also, hydrogenated vegetable fats such as those found in many margarines and processed foods should be avoided.

Dietary fats play a very important role in hormonal functioning as well. As a matter of fact, reproductive hormones cannot be made in adequate quantities if fat levels are too low. Sex hormones and adrenal hormones are actually made from the fat substance cholesterol. This does not mean that if a woman is in menopause she should start eating lots of cholesterol. It means that any woman who tends to restrict her fat and cholesterol intake severely, perhaps for weight control purposes, may not be able to manufacture optimal hormone levels as efficiently as she should.

Wheat Bran

Over the last several years there has been a movement toward eating more fibre to improve health and intestinal regularity. This is a very positive step and, no doubt, it has yielded many helpful results. Nevertheless, where osteoporosis is concerned it is very important to make sure that the type of fibre being consumed in large quantities is preferably *not* wheat-based.

It seems that wheat bran has the unfortunate attribute of binding with calcium and other bone-related minerals in the digestive tract, rendering them less absorbable. Switching to another form of fibre, at least when you have consumed higher amounts of calcium, is advisable if you are at risk of osteoporosis. These issues will be covered in more detail, in the 'Positive Foods' section below.

The foods that have been discussed so far represent the major dietary concerns related to menopause in general, as well as to osteoporosis. For many women, eating these foods in moderation rather than eliminating them completely from the diet may be adequate to avoid any major problems. For others, especially those with a higher risk of osteoporosis, or who already have hormonal or reproductive problems, a purposeful movement toward exclusion of the problem foods (and non-foods – alcohol, caffeine, etc.) may be advisable.

POSITIVE FOODS

While it is clear that many foods are better left alone during the menopause, conversely there are some that should be increased in the diet. Some of these foods may be beneficial because of some necessary substance they contain. Others may help to counteract an adverse effect of a negative food. Often, such foods offer a combination of these benefits.

Many nutrients derived from foods play a very important role in the production as well as in the balancing of the hormones of the endocrine system, such as those of the adrenal, hypothalamus and pituitary glands. Others, as you know, are essential for the health of the bones.

High-nutrient Diet

One of the key goals in setting up an appropriate diet for the menopausal years is to consume foods with the widest scope and highest levels of such nutrients. In general, the diet should be rich in all essential nutrients and fibre – with an emphasis on:

- the B vitamins, especially B_6 and pantothenic acid
- vitamin C
- the fat soluble vitamins, especially vitamins E and D and all essential minerals, especially calcium, magnesium, and zinc

Vegetables and Fruits

Vegetables and fruits represent rich sources of vitamins and minerals. Vegetables in particular are important as they contain many of the minerals notoriously lacking in the average Western diet, such as zinc and magnesium. They can also be a rich source of dietary calcium. Both vegetables and fresh fruits are generally high in nutrient value without being filled with a lot of negative attributes.

Other than the basic nutrient content of vegetables

and fruits, their dietary fibre content is one of their most beneficial aspects. As you may know, fibre (primarily the indigestible material in plants) has many benefits to the state of the intestinal tract. If the intestines are working properly, then the removal of harmful substances (including hormonal waste) is speeded up.

Whole Grains
Whole cereal grains – such as brown rice, oats, wheat, rye, barley, and corn – should also be plentiful in the diet of a menopausal or pre-menopausal woman. These foods are also extremely rich in essential nutrients. They are very high in B vitamins, many minerals, and essential fatty acids. Their nutrient and fibre content are also excellent, provided the grain is unrefined or processed. For instance, brown rice and whole wheat are excellent sources of fibre, while white rice and white flour (from wheat) are not, because in these latter grains the fibre and much of the nutritional value have been stripped away. Remember to concentrate less on wheat than the other grains due to the calcium-inhibiting effect of wheat bran. Exclusion should not be necessary however.

Beans/Legumes
Like whole grains, a diet high in beans or legumes provides a very rich source of nutritional value. As well as B vitamins and many minerals, these foods offer a good source of dietary protein with a far better calcium-to-phosphorus ratio than meat. Their fibre content is excellent and may aid in intestinal regularity, detoxification and blood sugar balance.

Fibre – Soluble versus Insoluble
The type of fibre that is of particular value in aiding the

detoxification of substances from the intestines is *soluble fibre*. This is the type of fibre that actually absorbs moisture, softens and swells in size. Soluble fibre is found in many foods – including brown rice, oats and apples (in the form of pectin). One of the more popular and useful forms that is being used in food supplements today is *psyllium seed husks*. These husks are preferable to the type of fibre found in whole wheat (bran), which is classed as *cellulose*. Cellulose is essentially insoluble and does not gel as does soluble fibre, although it does help remove solid waste from the intestines. Also, it is important to remember that wheat bran fibre is implicated in hindering the absorption of calcium.

As a rule, it would always be of value to help to maintain intestinal regularity by increasing dietary fibre in general; however, it would appear that forms of soluble fibre will accomplish this task as well as insoluble forms; forms of soluble fibre will also contribute their other valuable detoxifying and blood-sugar-regulating attributes and have less of a tendency to block calcium absorption. Because of its swelling or bulking properties, soluble fibre is also used by many to reduce hunger pangs (if taken with ample fluids prior to meals).

Dairy Products – Good or Bad?

It seems that many women have been encouraged – by friends, doctors and aggressive advertising campaigns – to increase their intake of dairy products significantly in order to improve bone health. Considering the rather high concentration of the mineral calcium in these foods, this would appear sound advice. Nevertheless, not all experts are so convinced. In order to find out why, let's examine a few of the relevant arguments for and against dairy foods.

MILK AND CALCIUM

Depending on which statistics you read, the amount of dietary calcium required per day by a menopausal woman may be in the range of 1,000 – 1,500 milligrams (mg). Some experts recommend even more.

There is no question that the calcium concentration in milk products is quite high and thus may be one of the more practical ways to achieve such levels. A cup of either whole, skimmed or low-fat milk contains close to a few hundred mg of calcium. Cheese is also a very concentrated source. There is a considerable down side, though.

As mentioned, calcium is not the only nutrient involved in bone structure. As a matter of fact, nutrients such as magnesium and vitamin D are essential in adequate quantities in order for calcium to carry out its function in the bones. If either of these nutrients is missing or deficient, then calcium will not be utilized properly. As a matter of fact, the more calcium being consumed, the more nutrients such as magnesium are needed. This is a factor not just in bone health but in the health of the other parts of the body where calcium and magnesium regulate physiological functions.

CALCIUM AND MAGNESIUM

The mineral magnesium is a constituent of bone. However, magnesium also has a mechanism that somehow helps with proper calcium utilization. (This will be explained in the next chapter.) Milk does contain small amounts of magnesium, but not in the appropriate balance that is required throughout the body.

About 99 per cent of the body's calcium is in the bones. A far lower percentage of magnesium levels is found in the bones. Much of the magnesium the body requires is needed in other cells, where, among other things, it helps to regulate nerve and muscle function as well as to aid energy production throughout the body. The amount of magnesium that is recommended is about half that of the calcium intake. As a result of this, the small amount of magnesium found in milk is very likely to be used up for these other, more pressing requirements to sustain life. Consequently, less will aid in bone development. Some possible answers to this dilemma will be explored in the next chapter.

FAT, CHOLESTEROL AND MILK

In the last section I discussed one of the more detrimental sides of milk products – the negative effect of saturated fats and cholesterol. This, however, is not a major concern for all women, although the risk of heart disease does increase as oestrogen levels lower with age. Fortunately, there are quite a few non-fat milk products available that would certainly help to reduce the threat of heart disease and other problems caused by too much of the wrong kind of fats.

Where cholesterol is concerned, the story is not so clear cut. It is now becoming clear that reducing cholesterol levels in the diet is by no means a guarantee that blood cholesterol levels will drop. Nevertheless, if you are at a higher risk of heart disease, whether menopausal or not it is advisable to be moderate with dietary cholesterol.

DAIRY INTOLERANCE

Dairy products and especially those from cow's milk can often produce either an allergic reaction or some form of intolerance. Much of the intolerance to cow's milk products is related to what is known as *lactose intolerance*. Lactose is a type of sugar found in milk which many people do not have the ability to adequately digest. Lactose intolerance results in digestive disturbances such as severe bloating, gas and diarrhoea. Statistics show that a rather high percentage of those who suffer with osteoporosis are lactose intolerant. Many people are sensitive to other constituents in milk rather than lactose.

Fatty Fish

While red meat may not be particularly suitable in large amounts for menopausal women, you do not have to be a vegetarian to be healthy at this time of life. As a matter of fact, there are attributes of certain types of fish that may be of great value.

FISH AND EPA

I have already discussed the negative effect that certain fatty substances can have on the body. There are, however, other types that can actually be beneficial. One such type is a fatty acid called eicosapentaenoic acid (EPA). EPA is primarily found in oily fish such as salmon, mackerel, sardines, cod and herring, among others. In order to get the best benefits from consuming fatty acids such as EPA in fish it is very important that the fish is *not* fried; preferably it should be cooked in the least 'aggressive' method possible (e.g. by poaching or steaming).

The effects of EPA are far too diverse to go into here, but one main benefit that this fatty acid possesses is in the area of circulation. EPA has an ability to reduce excessive blood clotting significantly, thereby improving circulation. This may be of great value in the menopause. Restricting certain types of fats while

increasing others is no guarantee that hot flushes and
night sweats will disappear, but anything that benefits
the circulation in general would be advisable.

Although yet to be confirmed by research other than
that performed on animals, EPA may have a protective
effect against breast cancer.

FISH AND VITAMIN D

Vitamin D is, of course, very important for the health of
the bones. Unfortunately it is extremely difficult to
obtain in the diet. Unless you consume foods that are
fortified with vitamin D (such as some dairy products),
the best food source of this elusive nutrient is certain
types of fish. The vitamin D in fish is primarily found in
their liver, although the flesh of tuna and herring
contain appreciable amounts. Vitamin D can be derived
from another source as well, which will be discussed in
the next chapter.

FISH AND THE PHOSPHORUS-TO-CALCIUM RATIO

Although the ratio of phosphorus to calcium in fish is
certainly not in favour of strong bones, it is not nearly
as bad as the 20:1 to 30:1 ratio found in red meat. The
content of vitamin D in certain fish also makes it a far
more acceptable source of non-vegetable protein.

Poultry

With regard to the phosphorus-to-calcium ratio, much
the same can be said of poultry – far less detrimental
than red meat, but not in the least beneficial for a
person's bone mineral profile.

The fat profile of poultry such as chicken and turkey
is preferable to that of red meat as well. It is considerably better to eat the white meat as opposed to the dark

meat, as the saturated fat and cholesterol content of the latter is far higher.

This chapter should give the menopausal woman some direction as to how to proceed from a dietary standpoint. As you might expect, the earlier you start with a proper dietary regime, the better. Hormonal and/or glandular disturbances do not occur overnight. The wrong type of eating (and drinking) habits over a matter of years can do untold damage to the endocrine system in general as well as to the reproductive system specifically. Even though the development of problems is not always dietary in origin, a poor diet will only make matters worse.

Just how far you should follow the above information is up to you. For many women moderation will be adequate, while for others a more strict approach might be warranted. Regardless of the issue of menopause, many of the facts in this chapter should help you to formulate a way of eating that is much healthier.

CHAPTER 7

Nutritional and Herbal Treatment of the Menopause and Osteoporosis

A sound dietary approach to the menopause is vital to reduce the adverse effects that can be experienced by many women at this time. It is never too late to gain at least some benefits from making adjustments to your diet; if the adjustments are consistent, especially over a period of time, the benefits may be substantial.

However, no matter how good your diet becomes, if you have not started making improvements until you are near to or have started the menopause, then there will be less chance of avoiding problems. This is especially true in the case of osteoporosis.

Since the malfunctions in the glandular system that predispose a woman to a more difficult menopause often start quite early in life, *this* should be the time when you start to eat healthily. After all, prevention is the only guaranteed way to cure anything. However, how many women are likely to try to avoid problems of the menopause while they are still in their twenties?

ADDRESSING THE CAUSE AS WELL AS THE SYMPTOMS

When treating any condition it is best not only to address its symptoms but also its cause. When we analyse the research into female hormonal problems it becomes quite clear that there are certain natural or non-drug substances that do reduce or correct many of the causes of symptoms as well as the symptoms themselves. While much of this research centres around premenstrual problems, more and more is focusing on the menopause and osteoporosis.

RENEWED HOPE THROUGH NUTRIENTS AND HERBS

Among the substances that have been proven to be beneficial are many vitamins and minerals. Other beneficial substances include amino acids, fatty acids, enzymes and herbs. One of the most valuable aspects of the results of research is that it has found that not only are these substances effective but that they can be so *without* the high risk of side-effects or toxicity.

A NEED FOR SUPPLEMENTATION

There exists a major limitation of dietary changes, aside from the fact that they are likely not to begin until a woman is experiencing menopause. While eating the right foods is a great way to avoid harmful substances, this does not often provide a woman with the *therapeutic* quantities of those nutrients that have been proven to benefit the symptoms and/or correct the causes of menopausal problems, including osteoporosis. Also, the therapeutic amounts of certain nutrients are limited as to what they can accomplish. In such cases, various herbal therapies may 'fill the gaps'.

Natural medicine has much to offer in the fight against so many different disorders. Fortunately, the medical and scientific journals are full of clinical trials and other research studies that prove the effectiveness and safety of many natural therapies. Lets look at some of the most useful and scientifically proven of the therapies used to treat menopausal symptoms and osteoporosis. They include vitamin and mineral supplementation, amino acid and enzyme therapy, and herbal medicine.

NUTRITIONAL AND HERBAL SUPPLEMENTATION

Calcium
The role of calcium cannot be overemphasized in terms of its importance in combating osteoporosis. As mentioned earlier, calcium is the most abundant mineral in bone tissue. Besides being so plentiful in bone, calcium also stimulates the release of the hormone calcitonin, which causes bone material to be deposited on the bones.

CALCIUM AND MILK
Much of the emphasis on calcium intake has focussed on the various sources of the mineral. Milk products have been the primary target of this emphasis, yet there are, of course, shortcomings to and controversies surrounding dairy products:

- They are too low in magnesium levels (it also appears that vitamin D-fortified dairy products reduce magnesium absorption).
- They can cause adverse (allergic/intolerance) reactions.
- They are often high in saturated fats and cholesterol.

Having said this, milk is nevertheless one of the most concentrated sources of calcium. The question remains, however: is the liberal intake of dairy products enough to create *adequate* calcium status? Theoretically it could be, at least as far as calcium intake itself is concerned. However, if you observe the statistics you find, for example, that the average daily intake of calcium in the US appears to be between 450 and 500 milligrams (mg) per person per day – compare this to the 1,000 to 1,500 mg per day menopausal and post-menopausal women should have to maintain good health. Nor does this take into account the other nutrients that are essential in order for calcium to benefit the bones in the first place, such as magnesium, zinc and vitamin D.

CALCIUM AND PHOSPHORUS

The other thing that must be considered when deciding how much calcium a menopausal woman needs is her intake of phosphorus.

The greater the phosphorus intake, the greater the calcium intake must be. Because the proportions in a typical 'Western' diet fall far too high on the phosphorus side, it is clear that there is the potential for real health problems here too.

Even the medical and pharmaceutical communities are resigning themselves to the overwhelming odds stacked against women in this area, and are looking to calcium supplementation to make up the difference.

CALCIUM RESEARCH

There is some evidence that increasing the intake of calcium reduces the incidence of bone loss; however, not all of the research studies were in agreement about this. In addition, some of the studies monitored dietary intake alone; others analysed the effects of calcium supplementation to the diet. Some very interesting observations arise upon deeper scrutiny of what the studies have discovered. Some of their more significant findings are as follows:

- A high calcium diet and/or a diet supplemented with calcium benefits many, but not all women.
- It was found in one study in which calcium supplements and sub-clinical hormone replacement were compared that each was effective in improving calcium balance. This prompted the suggestion that perhaps calcium supplementation should be considered a woman's first treatment, before HRT is implemented. Then, if the results of supplementation alone are not good after a period of time, hormone replacement could be utilized.
- Those who were supplemented with vitamin D as well as calcium fared better than those who used just one or the other.
- Different forms of calcium were shown to yield different results.

PROBLEMS WITH CALCIUM

If we know that calcium is so crucial for bone density, and we even have a good idea as to how much may be required, then why don't *all* women achieve positive results from a high calcium intake?

The answer to this question probably lies almost entirely within the third and fourth points above.

CALCIUM ABSORPTION

For a variety of reasons, it is often the case that the

body cannot absorb calcium adequately. Mineral absorption is a subject that requires its own book to explain, but suffice it to say that calcium is not very easy to absorb, particularly for women in their menopausal years. No matter how much calcium a person takes, he or she is not going to get the benefit of each and every mg ingested. This is due to the fact that the percentage of calcium that can be absorbed by the intestinal tract is far less than might be imagined. That which is not absorbed will have no benefit to the bones or any other part of the body.

DIGESTION AND CALCIUM

The first requirement that must be fulfilled in order for calcium to be absorbed is that it needs an acidic environment. This acidity is required to put calcium in what is known as a 'soluble' state. If this is not accomplished, then the calcium is unlikely to be absorbed in ample quantities.

This is particularly true in the case of calcium supplementation. Most calcium supplements on the market, such as *calcium carbonate*, are in an *in*soluble form. In order for the calcium to be absorbed it must first be separated from the carbonate compound it is bound to. If there is sufficient stomach acid (e.g. hydrochloric acid) at the time of ingestion, then more of the calcium will become soluble and easier to absorb. If the stomach acid is deficient, much of the calcium will be excreted and thus wasted.

STOMACH ACID AND MENOPAUSE

It has been found that women past the menopausal transition are much more likely to have exceedingly low levels of stomach acid. This would, of course, lead to much lower calcium absorption – in the women who need it the most. When calcium carbonate is used by those with ample stomach acid, the absorption rate of calcium is around 20 per cent of the total ingested amount. In those with low stomach acidity, this amount may be less than 5 per cent!

An absorption problem exists even in the case of food sources of calcium. Aside from weak digestion, many other factors can cause the calcium in food stuffs to be inadequately absorbed.

The statistics go a long way to explaining the inconsistent results obtained by women taking calcium. Obviously, then, the priorities for menopausal women are twofold. First, they should seek more easily soluble forms of calcium; secondly, they must address any digestion problems they might have. This second priority will be covered shortly.

OTHER FORMS OF CALCIUM

Besides the insoluble varieties (calcium carbonate, dolomite, etc.), fortunately there are other forms of calcium as well. The most absorbable are those that are chelated (bound) to organic acids, such as:

- calcium citrate
- amino acid chelated calcium
- calcium lactate
- calcium gluconate

CALCIUM CITRATE SUPERIORITY

One favourable outcome of the vast amount of research done on calcium and the menopause has been the discovery that certain forms of calcium can be absorbed *in spite of* the low stomach acidity found in many menopausal women. *Calcium citrate* is perhaps the best example of this. It seems that calcium citrate has three main attributes that make it so valuable:

1. It is already in a soluble and an organically chelated form.
2. According to research, women with low stomach acidity are still able to absorb perhaps over 40 per cent of the calcium in calcium citrate.
3. Calcium citrate has an exceedingly low risk of producing kidney stones. (Although rare, some susceptible individuals may develop calcium oxalate stones if ingesting high levels of calcium.)

Just how much can be gained if a woman does start taking calcium citrate while in her fifties or sixties depends on many factors:

- the absorbability of the calcium source being used
- the quantity being taken
- the state of the woman's bones at the time
- the existence of other nutrients required for healthy bones
- the strength of the woman's digestive system
- her unique biochemistry

Perhaps the best time to start addressing osteoporosis is when a woman is in her twenties rather than her fifties, but any time is better than never at all. Provided the form of calcium being utilized is more readily absorbable, then there may still be great benefits to be had in preventing or slowing further bone loss. There may even be increased bone density over a long period of time.

DOSAGE

The dosage requirement varies from woman to woman. Research seems to indicate a daily intake of about 1,000 to 1,500 mg per day. Pre-menopausal women may be able to stick to the lower end of this range; post-menopausal women may want to take the higher dosage.

Of course, even if a woman's intake of calcium is more than adequate, and even if the form used is easily absorbed, there is still a need for certain other nutrients to be available in ample quantities.

Vitamin D

Vitamin D is sometimes considered a hormone rather than a vitamin. One of its primary roles in the body is to trigger absorption of calcium in the small intestine. It seems to do this by stimulating the production of a certain protein molecule in the intestinal wall which attaches to calcium, thereby aiding in its journey into the blood.

SOURCES OF VITAMIN D

As mentioned before, vitamin D is very difficult to get in the diet, especially if fish or vitamin D-fortified dairy products are not eaten regularly. Fortunately we do produce vitamin D ourselves, without ever having to consume it.

Vitamin D is manufactured in our bodies from the action of ultraviolet (UV) rays on the cholesterol in our skin. Whether or not this is adequate to prevent osteoporosis depends on the individual as well as on the length of time the skin surface is exposed to UV light.

Vitamin D supplements, should they be required, will be derived from the liver oil of some types of fish (e.g.

cod liver oil), although some non-fish sources (e.g. sheep's wool and yeast irradiation) are also available.

DOSAGE

Vitamin D is classified as a fat-soluble vitamin and thus has the capability to be stored in the liver until it is required. As a result, large amounts are not generally required on a frequent basis. Many multiple-vitamin formulas contain reasonable amounts of this nutrient. Such amounts and some UV exposure may be all that a woman requires to maintain adequate levels of vitamin D in her system. However, occasionally separate supplementation is needed.

The levels used are generally between 300 and 400 iu. Levels far in excess of this (i.e. over 3,000 iu per day) may cause side-effects such as an overabundance of calcium in certain parts of the body, and is therefore not recommended.

Magnesium

A deficiency in the mineral magnesium has been noted in osteoporotic people. Even though the amount of magnesium found in the bones is far less than that of calcium, it appears to play an absolutely essential role in bone health.

In a roundabout way, magnesium induces the re-absorption of calcified bone. Magnesium may also be useful in preventing the excessive accumulation of calcium in the wrong parts of the body, such as the kidneys. On the other hand, too little magnesium leads to lower levels of the most active form of vitamin D (called 1,25 dihydroxycholecalciferol).

OTHER BENEFITS

Aside from its effects on calcium, magnesium helps to regulate the functioning of the nerves, which could be very helpful during the menopause. For those women who are pre-menopausal and still menstruating, magnesium supplementation has been proven to reduce significantly several premenstrual symptoms such as nervous tension, general aches and pains, breast pain and excessive premenstrual weight gain. Magnesium is also one of the most protective nutrients for the cardio-vascular system.

DOSAGE

The magnesium levels in the bone are far lower than those of calcium. However, due to the many roles this mineral plays in other parts of the body, the requirement needed cannot be gauged based on bone content alone. It is often recommended that magnesium should be consumed in quantities that are about half those of calcium. Each person's needs may vary for different reasons, but this is the rule of thumb. If the levels of calcium consumed are 1,000 mg per day, then the magnesium intake would be about 500 mg.

SOURCES

Many calcium supplements also contain magnesium, often in the advised 2 to 1 proportion. As with calcium, it is best that the magnesium is consumed in any easily soluble form. Some good dietary sources of magnesium include dark green vegetables, whole grains and almonds.

Boron

The trace mineral boron has been the subject of some

very interesting research of late. There are two main ways in which boron may be vital for menopausal women: in its effect on oestrogen levels and bone density.

Research has shown that the supplementation of boron caused an increased activity of one of the forms of oestrogen (*oestradiol*) in post-menopausal women. Boron also seems to increase the retention of bone-related minerals such as calcium and magnesium. At least part of this effect may be due to the positive influence of boron on vitamin D activity.

DOSAGE
It would appear from the research that 3 mg of boron per day is probably adequate to reap its benefits.

SOURCES
Fresh vegetables and fruits are good sources of this mineral. If supplementation is used, the boron should be in an organically chelated form.

Silicon
Another trace mineral, *silicon*, may also play a major role in protection against osteoporosis. While boron appears to be involved more in the mechanics behind bone building, silicon seems to play a substantial role in the bone tissue itself.

Also referred to as *silica*, silicon is a necessary element of human connective tissue. This makes it very important in the building of strong skin, hair, nails, blood vessels, etc. Silicon also seems to provide the substance needed to manufacture the 'glue' that holds bone tissue together.

DOSAGE

Although an official requirement has not yet been established, many experts suggest that all adults should take somewhere between 20 and 25 mg per day.

SOURCES

The richest sources of silicon are various plant fibres such as those found in whole brown rice and oats. Alfalfa is also a good source of this trace element.

A few different forms of silicon are used as supplements. A common source is derived from sand (silicon dioxide). Preferable alternatives include the herb *horsetail* (*equisetum arvense*) and a red algae called *lithothamnium calcareum*. The algae form is often used in order to avoid the considerable diuretic effect of horsetail.

The nutrients discussed above represent some of the primary substances the body needs to maintain proper bone density. Ensuring an adequate intake of these and of the nutrients and herbs that follow may greatly aid in preventing the development of osteoporosis and/or helping to treat it once it has begun.

Vitamin E

One of the most well known of the family of vitamins is *vitamin E*. Vitamin E carries out many different processes in the body. One of the most relevant to the needs of the menopausal woman is its positive effect on the circulatory system.

VITAMIN E AND HOT FLUSHES

Among the most common of all menopausal symptoms are hot flushes and night sweats. These symptoms are caused when a defect (often referred to as 'vasomotor dysfunction') occurs in the normal functioning of certain blood vessels. When a woman experiences a hot flush, the blood vessels allow an unusually heavy rush of blood to the surface of the uppermost portion of her body. This produces the rise in local temperature and the flushing.

EARLY CLINICAL TRIALS

Oestrogen supplementation has been a common drug treatment for menopausal vasomotor symptoms for decades. As far back as the mid-1940s, however, there was clinical evidence that vitamin E worked – and generally without associated side-effects! We may think of the research into natural medicine as being a fairly recent phenomenon but, as a matter of fact, by 1952 there had already been a few studies performed and published in medical journals demonstrating vitamin E's unquestionable success.

Vitamin E has long been known for its positive effects on the blood vessels, circulation and the cardiovascular system in general. These effects include, among other things, reducing excessive blood clotting. Where hot flushes are concerned, vitamin E seems to correct the vasomotor dysfunction that causes hot flushes.

OTHER BENEFITS

Hot flushes and night sweats are not the only symptoms that may benefit greatly from vitamin E supplementation. In some of the earliest clinical trials using only vitamin E, many menopausal symptoms were noticeably diminished or even eliminated, including:

- hot flushes
- night sweats
- fatigue

- dizziness
- heart palpitations
- muscle, joint and backaches and pain
- nervous tension
- some symptoms associated with pre-menopausal menstruation

Quite an impressive list for one vitamin! In these early trials, results were often obtained fairly quickly (from within a few weeks to a few months), the potencies used varying from experiment to experiment. At this time it appears that vitamin E should be a major part of the natural treatment of menopausal symptoms.

DOSAGE
Daily intake will depend on the individual, but it would appear that between 200 and 600 iu per day should be appropriate for most women. If a woman has high blood pressure, it may be best to start with the lower amount and gradually increase as and if necessary.

SOURCES
Vitamin E supplementation can be used, as well as generally eating more of the foods that contain vitamin E, such as raw vegetable oils, raw seeds and nuts, wheat germ and soybeans.

B Vitamins
Many of the *B-complex* family of vitamins may play an important role in the menopause as well. The B–complex is made up of several different nutrients, known as B vitamins. Each has its own effects on the body, many of which are relevant to the menopause, and its symptoms, as well as osteoporosis.

Pantothenic acid (vitamin B$_5$) is often called the 'anti-stress nutrient'. Many nutrients have a positive effect on stress, but pantothenic acid is among the more important. Pantothenic acid is among the main nutrients needed in order to manufacture adrenal hormones.

It has been found that when pantothenic acid levels are inadequate, the adrenal glands may atrophy. This, of course, would not only lead to lower stress tolerance but also to exhaustion and other characteristics of low adrenal hormone output. Also, if the adrenal glands are weakened in this manner this would presumably affect the production of adrenal oestrogen (so important during and after menopause).

Folic acid and *vitamin B$_6$ (pyridoxine)* are needed in order for the non-mineral matrix of the bone to be manufactured properly. In addition, research suggests that B$_6$ may be useful in relieving many of the symptoms of premenstrual tension.

Other members of the B-complex family may be of use as well; those mentioned above are just a few of the more relevant ones.

DOSAGE AND SOURCES

Individual requirements for each of the B vitamins vary. Many people choose to take a supplement of the B-complex, where several different B vitamins are found together. An average of about 50 mg per day of most of the B vitamins, as contained in such a supplement, is probably appropriate (with the exception of folic acid and *biotin*, which are generally found in microgram [mcg] dosages.) Certain multiple vitamin/mineral formulas will contain similar levels of the B complex as well.

Dietary sources include brown rice and other whole grains, brewer's yeast, and liver.

L-tyrosine

Another substance that can be of great value in combating the symptoms of the menopause is the amino acid *l-tyrosine*. Amino acids are the components used to make proteins in the body. There are many different amino acids and each affects the body differently. One of the major effects of l-tyrosine happens to be particularly relevant to the menopause.

FUNCTIONS

Clinical studies have uncovered one l-tyrosine's more useful actions in the body. Due to the fact that it increases levels of certain chemicals in the brain, l-tyrosine has been shown in research to have anti-depressive effects. This, of course, could be of great use to many menopausal women.

DOSAGE AND SOURCES

The amounts of l-tyrosine can vary in order to give an adequate effect. L-tyrosine can be made in the body from the amino acid *l-phenylalanine* (found in protein foods such as meat and dairy products), but for therapeutic purposes supplementation is generally required. If such supplementation is needed, it may be advised in levels between 250 mg and 500 mg per day.

It is clear that many nutrients have a great deal to offer in controlling menopausal symptoms. Another area of natural medicine that holds great promise is herbal therapy. There are many herbs that may be of value during the menopause and the later stages of the menstrual years; we will focus on one in particular – dong quai.

Dong Quai

The Chinese herb *dong quai* (*angelica sinensis*) is among the most revered herbs used in the treatment of disorders of the female reproductive system. Based on the research carried out, there appears to be great justification for its high stature. There are several different beneficial effects that dong quai seems to have on a woman's body.

FUNCTIONS

Hormone Balance

Dong quai appears to fit into a category of plants that can help to influence oestrogen levels. Such plants are thought to exert oestrogenic activity due to their content of what are known as phytoestrogens. Although the activity of phytoestrogens compared to that of oestrogen is far less potent, they nevertheless may have a beneficial effect on many of the symptoms associated with low oestrogen levels. On the other hand, if oestrogen levels are too high, as is often the case premenstrually, phytoestrogens can compete with oestrogen thereby reducing the side-effects associated with high oestrogen levels. This may help to explain one reason that taking phytoestrogens does not appear to cause the type of side-effects oestrogen replacement can bring on. This 'balancing effect' may account for some of the helpful activity associated with dong quai.

Regulating Menstruation

Dong quai has been used for centuries to help to regulate menstruation and menstrual flow and lessen period pain. Obviously these are positive influences, particularly so during the pre-menopausal phase when periods can be quite erratic and uncomfortable. This is not to say that dong quai will counteract the normal changes in the menstrual periods common to the menopausal transition; however, in some women it may be of use in reducing the severe fluctuations sometimes experienced. These regulating actions may be related to dong quai's modifying effect on uterine contractions and circulation, as noted in research, as well as any effect on hormonal regulation.

Soothing the Nervous System
Research has shown dong quai to have a relaxing effect on the central nervous system. This may be of value in reducing irritability, nervous tension and insomnia, all of which are associated with the menopause and PMT.

Analgesic Effect
Dong quai has a proven value in the reduction of many forms of chronic pain, including neuralgia and arthritis. Minor aches and pains are not uncommon in menopausal women.

Improving Circulation
Studies suggest that dong quai may have an ability to enhance circulation. It has been reported that dong quai may correct symptoms caused by a vitamin E deficiency.

At this time, it is doubtful that there is research to support all of the many claims made about dong quai in traditional Chinese medicine; nevertheless, research into herbal medicine is on the increase and even the data currently existing on dong quai is very encouraging.

See the list at the end of this chapter for suggested dosage levels of dong quai.

Vitamin C and Bioflavonoids

FUNCTIONS

In addition to its more well-known effects on the immune system, *vitamin C* is also needed to produce collagen. Collagen is a major constituent of bone tissue.

Bioflavonoids are plant-derived pigmenting agents. Many bioflavonoids have been found to strengthen collagen-based structures and thus may be of great value in improving the integrity of the non-mineral matrix of the bones.

Also, a very interesting study found that bio-flavonoids (from citrus) were beneficial in relieving menopausal vasomotor symptoms (such as hot flushes).

DOSAGE

Requirements do vary, but 500 to 1,500 mg of vitamin C per day and 100 to 500 mg of citrus bioflavonoids per day may be appropriate.

SOURCES

Many vitamin C supplements also contain bioflavonoids, as bioflavonoids appear to increase the activity of vitamin C in the body. Common dietary sources include fresh fruits and vegetables.

The above list represents some of the more effective, safe and research-proven nutritional and herbal supplements that can be used in the treatment of menopausal symptoms and the prevention of osteoporosis. There are many others that may be of value as well, but these are among the most useful.

Treatment Programme

The list that follows represents a hypothetical supplemental programme utilizing medically and scientifically researched substances for the natural treatment of menopausal symptoms and the prevention of osteoporosis. This information is *not* intended to be prescriptive and you should consult a qualified medical health practitioner before beginning any such programme.

For Menopausal Symptoms and Osteoporosis

Avoid or reduce the intake of:

- alcohol
- caffeine
- tobacco
- refined sugar
- soft drinks
- red meat
- fried foods and hydrogenated fats

Hypothetical recommendations

- vitamin E (200–600 IU daily)
- calcium citrate (800–1,000 mg daily)
- magnesium citrate (400–500 mg daily) (calcium and magnesium can often be found together in the same formula)
- boron – chelated (3 mg daily)
- silicon (20–25 mg daily)
- dong quai (500–1,000 mg daily)
- vitamin C 500–1,500 mg with bioflavonoids 100–500 mg daily)
- multiple vitamin/mineral (with minimum 40–50 mg B-complex, vitamin D, and 10–15 mg of zinc) as directed on label

Optional
- l-tyrosine (250–500 mg daily – not to be taken at same time as high-protein foods

CHAPTER 8

Putting Knowledge into Action

It is unfortunate that at this time much of the available information on treating and preventing health disorders never reaches the people who need it most – sufferers. Nevertheless, it can be comforting to know that there continues to be important and impressive research on many such subjects, including the menopause and osteoporosis. It may be even more comforting to know that much of this research involves the use of natural medicine.

It has been the intention of this book to give you a comprehensive account of the current data on the menopause and osteoporosis, their treatment and/or (in the case of osteoporosis) prevention. This way you can make the most informed choices about the available methods of natural treatment available.

WEIGHING THE OPTIONS

You should never go into any treatment programme without understanding the positive and negative aspects as best as possible. Even though menopause itself is not a health disorder it is no exception to this rule. Everyone is different, and thus the modes of treatment may differ from person to person. The effectiveness and, in some cases, the likelihood of side-effects may vary as well. This has certainly been highlighted in the case of hormone replacement therapy (HRT).

Where a natural therapy such as nutritional and herbal medicine is concerned, the effectiveness of many substances is often incredibly high while the risk of side-effects or toxicity is extremely low. This generally allows such programmes to be infinitely more flexible than those utilizing drugs. The effects of any natural therapy can vary somewhat as well, however, and you should not go into such a programme without first understanding what it entails.

The method of therapy you choose does not have to be an 'all or nothing' decision. There are many women who may choose to utilize both a natural programme as well as the standard medical approach.

For various reasons, many women may be adverse to the idea of HRT. As a result, once they are aware of non-drug methods which can be used, many consider discontinuing HRT. This is especially the case when a woman has experienced unpleasant side-effects caused by the oestrogen drug. While this is understandable, *never* discontinue HRT without first consulting your doctor.

DIETARY CHANGES ARE VITAL

Once a person knows that there are nutritional and herbal supplements that may be very potent in correcting or reducing a disorder, they might feel they should use the supplements *instead* of following other dietary advice. While many supplements may be of great value regardless of diet, best results will most likely be achieved by using supplements *and* maintaining a healthy diet.

It is important to remember that many foods (or non-foods) can do untold damage to the hormones and the bones. Making the suggested dietary changes, or at least moving in that direction, could significantly reduce the chance of further damage to the body. This applies not only to problems associated with the menopause. Many substances discussed under 'Negative Foods' in Chapter Six are also negative factors in the development and/or worsening of several different health disorders in women and men.

As mentioned earlier, for some women moderation of these negative foods may be adequate. For those in more severe circumstances, however, perhaps complete avoidance of these foods should be the aim.

The Power of Supplementation

While dietary changes are indeed vital, the foods you eat, whether good or bad, often lack the potency of nutrients needed in the treatment of the menopause and osteoporosis. As a result, many women have found using supplements a great benefit. Herbal therapies have been found to fill the treatment gaps left by certain nutrients. This is an increasingly important area of research and offers exciting prospects above and beyond that which have already been proven.

A UNIFIED APPROACH

It is clear that a unified approach to the menopause and its associated problems may offer women the best help. Research also points to the fact that lifestyle improvements such as regular exercise may further aid the dietary and supplement therapy, especially in fighting and/or preventing osteoporosis.

HOPE FOR THE FUTURE

Menopause is a very personal subject and each woman must decide for herself on the most appropriate approach for her needs. It is never too late to take responsibility for your health. Often the will is there but the information is lacking. Fortunately this is changing, and the scientific and medical research proving the benefits of natural medicine has provided the menopausal woman with a very valuable tool for improving her situation. Thanks to this information, relief of menopausal problems and suffering may be in your grasp!

BIBLIOGRAPHY

Abbey, L. *Journal of Orthomolecular Psychiatry*, 11, 1982, pp. 243–59.

Albanese, A. *et al. Nutrition Reports International*, 33, 6, 1986, pp. 879–91.

Alberti, K. & Natrass, M. *The Lancet*, 2, 1977, pp. 25–9.

Allen, G. *et al, American Journal of Clinical Nutrition*, 32, 1979, pp. 741–9.

Anderson, M. *et al. Journal of Nutrition*, 107, 1977, p. 834.

Baker, M. *et al. British Medical Journal*, 3 March, 1979, p. 589.

Bensky, D. & Gamble, A. *Chinese Herbal Medicine: Materia Medica*, Eastland Press, 1986.

Bickle, D. *et al. Annals of Internal Medicine*, 103, 1985, pp. 42–8.

British Medical Association. *Guide to Medicines and Drugs*, Dorling Kindersley, 1991.

Brooks, A. *Journal of Reproductive Medicine*, 26, 1981, p. 279.

Buist, R. *International Clinical Nutrition Review*, 5, 1985, pp. 1–4.

Caniggia, A. *et al. ACTA Vitaminology and Enzymology*, 6, 1984, pp. 117–30.

Canigglia, A. *et al. Journal of Endocrinal Invest.*, 7, 4, 1984, pp. 373–8.

Carlisle, E. *Science*, 167, Jan. 16, 1970, pp. 279–80.

Christy, C. *American Journal of Obstetrics and Gynacology*, 50, 1945, p. 84.

Cohen, L. & Kitzes, R. *Israeli Journal of Medical Science*, 17, 1981, pp. 1,123–5.

Deugun, M & Cohen, C. *American Journal of Clinical Nutrition*, 34, 1981, p. 1,501.

Draper, H. & Scythes, C. *Federation Proceedings*, 40, 9, 1981, pp. 2,434–8.

Ed. 'Citrate for calcium nephrolithiasis', *The Lancet*, i, 1986, p. 955.

Elghamry, M. & Shihata, I. *Planta Medica*, 13, 1965, pp. 352–7.

Ellis, F. *et al. American Journal of Clinical Nutrition*, 25, 1972, pp. 55–8.

Finkler, R. *Journal of Clinical Endocrinology and Metabolism*, 9, 1949, pp. 89–94.

Gallagher, J. *et al. Journal of Clinical Invest.*, 64, 1979, p. 729.

Gibson, C. & Gelenberg, A. *Advanced Biol. Psychiat.*, 10, 1983, pp. 148–59.

Goldberg, I. (letter to the editor), *The Lancet*, 2, 1980, p. 364.

Greden, J. *American Journal of Psychiatry*, Oct, 1974.

Harju, E. *et al. Archives in Orthopedic*

and Trauma Surgery, 103, 6, 1985, pp. 408–16.

Heaney, R. & Recker, R. *Journal of Laboratory and Clinical Medicine,* 99, 1982, pp. 46–55.

Heaney, R. *Clin. Invest. Medicine,* 5, 1981, pp. 147–55.

Heaney, R. & Recker, R. *American Journal of Clinical Nutrition,* 43, 1966, pp. 299–305.

Hill, P. & Wynder, E. *American Journal of Clinical Nutrition,* 33, 1980, p. 1,192.

Hollingbery, P. *et al. Federation Proceedings,* 44, 1985, p. 1,149.

Horowitz, M. *et al. American Journal of Clinical Nutrition,* 39, 1984, pp. 857–9.

Hussey, H. *Journal of the American Medical Association,* 235, 1976, p. 1,367.

Jick, H. *et al, The Lancet,* 14 April, 1977, p. 1,345.

Kavinoky, N. *Annals of Western Medicine and Surgery,* 4, 1, 1950, pp. 27–32.

Krasinski, S. *et al. Nutrition Today,* Jan/Feb 1988, pp. 4–7.

Krolner, B. *et al. Clinical Science,* 64, 1983, pp. 541–6.

Lee, C. *et al, American Journal of Clinical Nutrition,* 34, 1981, pp. 819–23.

Leung, A. *Encyclopedia of Common Natural Ingredients Used in Food, Drugs and Cosmetics,* John Wiley & Sons, 1980.

Licata, A. *American Journal of Clinical Nutrition,* 34, 1981, p. 1,779.

Lutz, J & Linkswiter, H. *American Journal of Clinical Nutrition,* 34, 1981, p. 2,178.

MacLennan, W. & Hamilton, J. *British Medical Journal,* 2, 1 Oct., 1977, pp. 859–61.

MacMahon, B. *et al. New England Journal of Medicine,* 307, 1982, p. 1,062.

Manthey, J. *Circulation,* 64, Oct, 1981, pp. 722–9.

Marcus, R. *Metabolism,* 31, 1982, pp. 93–102.

Marsh, A. *et al. American Journal of Clinical Nutrition,* 37, 1983, pp. 453–6.

Massey, L. & Berg, T. *Nutrition Research,* 5, 1985, pp. 1,281–4.

Mazzaferri, E. *Textbook of Endocrine Physiology* (3rd ed.), Elsevier Science Pub., 1986.

Moore, K. *Clinically Oriented Anatomy* (3rd ed.), Williams & Wilkins, 1992.

Murray, M. & Pizzorno, J. *Encyclopedia of Natural Medicine,* Macdonald and Co., 1990, pp. 461–2.

Newcomer, A. *et al. Annals of Internal Medicine,* 89, 1978, pp. 218–20.

Nicar, M. & Pak, C. *Journal of Clinical Endocrinology and Metabolism,* 61, 1985, pp. 91–393.

Nielson, F. *et al. Faseb. J.,* Feb. 15, 1989.

NIH Consensus Conference. *Journal of the American Medical Association,* 252, 6, 1984, pp. 782–799.

Nordin, B. *et al. American Journal of Clinical Nutrition,* 42, 3, 1985, pp. 470–74.

Parish, P. *Medical Treatments: The Benefits and Risks,* Penguin, 1991.

Passwater, R. and Cranton, E. *Trace Elements, Hair Analysis and Nutrition,* Keats, 1983.

Rainey, J. *et al. Psychopharmacology Bulletin,* 20, 1, 1984, pp. 45–9.

Recker, R. *New England Journal of Medicine,* 313, 1985, pp. 70–73.

Saville, P. *Journal of Bone and Joint Surgery,* 47a, 1965, pp. 492–9.

Schauf, C. *et al. Human Physiology*,
  Times Mirror/Mosby, 1990.
Seelig, M. *Cardiovascular Medicine*,
  3, 1978, pp. 637–50.
Smith, C. *Chicago Med.*, March 7, 1964.
Spencer, H. *et al. American Journal
  of Medicine*, 37, 1964, p. 223.
Steiner, M. *Thromb. Haemost.*, 49, 2,
  1983, pp. 73–7.

Thalassinos, N. *et al, Clinical Science*,
  62, 2, 1982, pp. 221–6.
Thom, J. *et al. British Journal of
  Urology*, 50, 1978, pp. 459–64.
Trowell, H. *American Journal of
  Clinical Nutrition*, 29, 1976,
  pp. 417–27.
Winick, M. *Nutritional Disorders of
  American Women*, Wiley, 1977.

INDEX